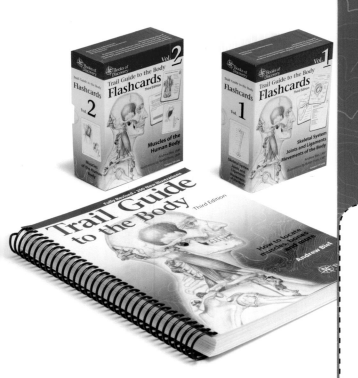
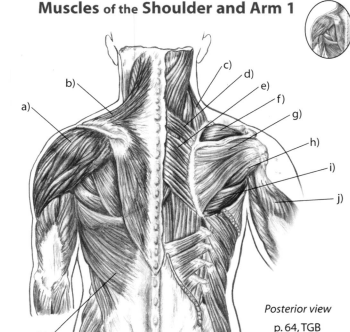
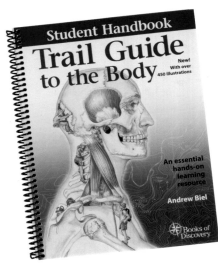
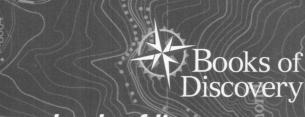

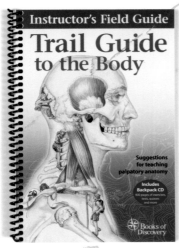

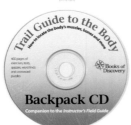

Instructor's Field Guide and Backpack (Quiz and Test Bank) CD:
In response to instructor requests, we created this 152-page Field Guide to assist teachers who are using *Trail Guide* in the classroom. Whether you are a new instructor, an experienced instructor looking for fresh ideas, or are just becoming familiar with *Trail Guide to the Body*, this will be an invaluable resource for you. This Field Guide follows the chapters and structures in *Trail Guide*, providing you with an easy-to-follow template and optional teaching elements.

The Instructor's Backpack CD (included with the Instructor's Field Guide) is stuffed with quizzes, fill-in illustrations, take-home assignments, word finds, crossword puzzles and more! 400+ pages, 850 illustrations. These items are FREE to institutions that require the *Trail Guide to the Body* textbook!

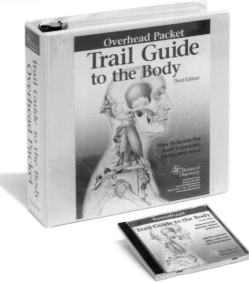

Visual Aids: Available in PowerPoint or Overhead format, these products feature illustrations and text to assist instructors in the hands-on, kinesthetic part of class. The Overhead Packet contains 750 illustrations on 234 transparencies. The PowerPoint features more than 900 illustrations on 500 slides.

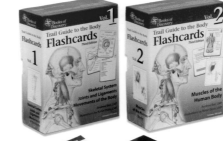

Textbook/Student Handbook/Flashcard Set Combo:
Purchase the 3rd Edition of the *Trail Guide to the Body* textbook and get 15% off the Student Handbook and the Volume I and Volume II flashcards. Available for U.S. retail customers only.

Textbook/Flashcard Set Combo:
Purchase the 3rd Edition of the *Trail Guide to the Body* textbook and get 15% off the Volume I and Volume II flashcards. Available for U.S. retail customers only.

Textbook/Handbook Combo:
Purchase the 3rd Edition of the *Trail Guide to the Body* textbook and get 15% off the Student Handbook. Available for U.S. retail customers only.

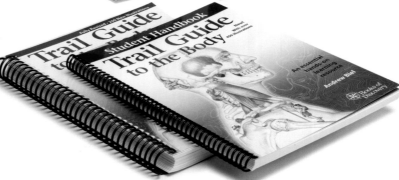

To order call 800-775-9227 or order online at www.booksofdiscovery.com

Visit our website for samples of all of our products.
Wholesale discounts are available. See our website or call for pricing.

International Distributors

United Kingdom/Europe
Ultimate Massage Solutions
www.ultimatemassagesolutions.com
44(0)7774 183458
info@ultimatemassagesolutions.com

Canada
Curties-Overzet Publications, Inc.
www.curties-overzet.com
1-888-649-5411 • info@curties-overzet.com

Australia and New Zealand
Akasha Books Limited - New Zealand
www.akasha.co.nz • info@akasha.co.nz
0800 252-742 (NZ) 64-4-296-1551 (AUS)

Trail Guide to the Body
How to locate muscles, bones and more

Student Handbook

First Edition

Andrew Biel, LMP
Licensed Massage Practitioner

Illustrations by Robin Dorn, LMP
Licensed Massage Practitioner

First Edition

Published by Books of Discovery
2539 Spruce St., Boulder, CO 80302 USA
www.booksofdiscovery.com
info@booksofdiscovery.com
800.775.9227

Associate Editors
Shelly Barnard
Dana Ecklund

Special thanks to Aaron Adams, Ashley Bechel, Miranda Legge,
Christine Malles, Gene Martinez and Mindy Morton.

Printed in Canada by Printcrafters, Winnipeg

Library of Congress Cataloging-in-Publication Data

Biel, Andrew R.
Trail Guide to the Body: Student Handbook
First Edition

ISBN: 978-0-9658534-6-0
Library of Congress Control Number: 2005902120

15 14 13 12 11 10 9 8 7

Disclaimer
The purpose of Books of Discovery's products is to provide
information for hands-on therapists on the subject of palpatory
anatomy. This book does not offer medical advice to the reader
and is not intended as a replacement for appropriate health-
care and treatment. For such advice, readers should consult
a licensed physician.

✵ Table of Contents

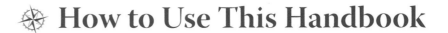

❋ How to Use This Handbook

Welcome to the *Trail Guide to the Body* Student Handbook. We designed this tool to help you develop and refine the techniques you have become familiar with in *Trail Guide* (3rd Edition).

You can find the answers at the back of the handbook, and each answer is followed by the page number that corresponds to information in *Trail Guide*.

The **red oval** at the top of each page also provides the page number that you can refer to in *Trail Guide* for more information.

In the **CHOICES** box, a number after the choice indicates how many locations on the illustration it can be used.

Many of the anatomy illustrations have been left **uncolored** so you can learn their structures by highlighting them with colored markers.

The **Shorten or Lengthen?** section is designed to help you learn the span of a muscle when a joint is in a specific position. If you become confused, try standing up and performing the movement on your own body. (There's nothing like a little kinesthetic exploration to help you find the answer.)

The **Let's Palpate!** section can get you started as you create your own palpatory journal (see pg. 19 in *Trail Guide*). Find three people - roommate, classmate, friend - and explore the specified bony landmark or muscle. Remember: There are no wrong answers, so you can describe what you feel in any way you prefer.

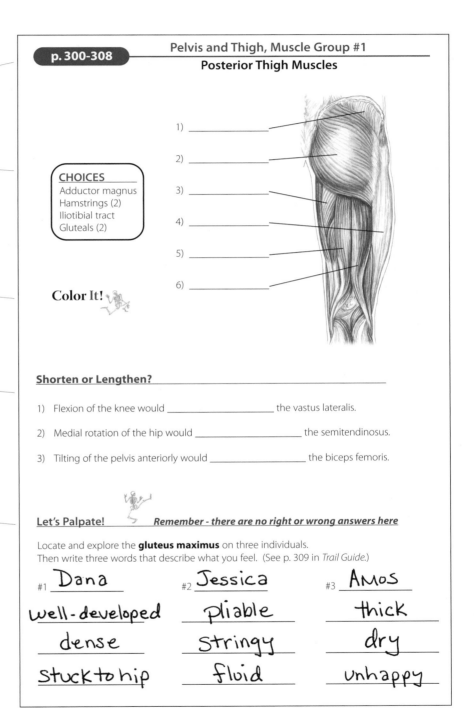

Hey, before you go: Those answer pages might be tempting, but try to use them only after you have completed the page or when you are really stuck. Happy trails!

Introduction
Tour Guide Tips #1

Please answer the following questions.

1) What are the "trail markers" that will help you locate muscles and tendons? _____

2) Since there are different body types and the terrain is never the same, explain how one "body map" could apply to all of them.

_____

3) What does "palpation" mean? _____

4) Palpation is an art and skill that involves _____ a structure, becoming

_____ of its characteristics and _____ its quality or condition.

5) Laying one hand on the other allows the bottom hand to stay receptive while the top hand

_____ and _____.

6) Name three ways palpation can be made easier by "working smart." _____

_____   _____

7) When outlining the shape or edge of a bone, it is best to roll your fingers _____ rather

than _____ its surface.

8) If the structure you are palpating is moving, your hands should _____.

9) When a movement is performed by your partner it is called _____ and when your partner

relaxes and allows you to do the movement it is called _____.

10) In *Trail Guide to the Body*, resisted movements are used to distinguish the _____,

_____ and _____ of different muscles and tendons.

11) As you improve your palpatory skills, what are three qualities or principles you will want to practice?

_____   _____   _____

12) Skeletal muscle is composed of nerves, blood vessels, _____ and _____.

13) A muscle's connective tissue layers merge at either end of the muscle to form a strong _____.

1) The muscle that carries out an action is called the _____, while the muscle that resists this action is the _____.

2) Please name the three physical characteristics which help to distinguish muscle from other tissues.

_____   _____   _____

3) To distinguish a tendon from a ligament, explore its _____ and _____.

4) Name three types of connective tissue that are palpable.

_____   _____   _____

5) Fascia is a continuous sheet of _____ located beneath the _____ and around muscles and organs.

6) A sharp, shooting sensation felt locally or down the corresponding appendage during palpation may be caused by _____.

Matching

Please match the term to the best definition.

1) _____ adipose
2) _____ aponeurosis
3) _____ artery
4) _____ bone
5) _____ bursa
6) _____ fascia
7) _____ ligament
8) _____ lymph node
9) _____ muscle
10) _____ nerve
11) _____ retinaculum
12) _____ skin
13) _____ tendon
14) _____ vein

a) a voluntary contractile tissue that moves the skeleton
b) two types - superficial and deep
c) a vessel easily seen on the dorsal surface of the hand
d) a vessel in which a pulse can be felt
e) a small, fluid-filled sac that reduces friction between two structures
f) a broad, flat tendon
g) a structure connecting bones together at a joint
h) easy to distinguish by its solid feel
i) bean-shaped ranging in size from pea to almond-sized
j) a tube-shaped vessel that becomes tender when compressed
k) a transverse thickening of deep fascia, strapping down tendons
l) the largest organ in the body
m) attaches muscle to bone
n) tissue with a gelatinous consistency

Please identify the following structures.

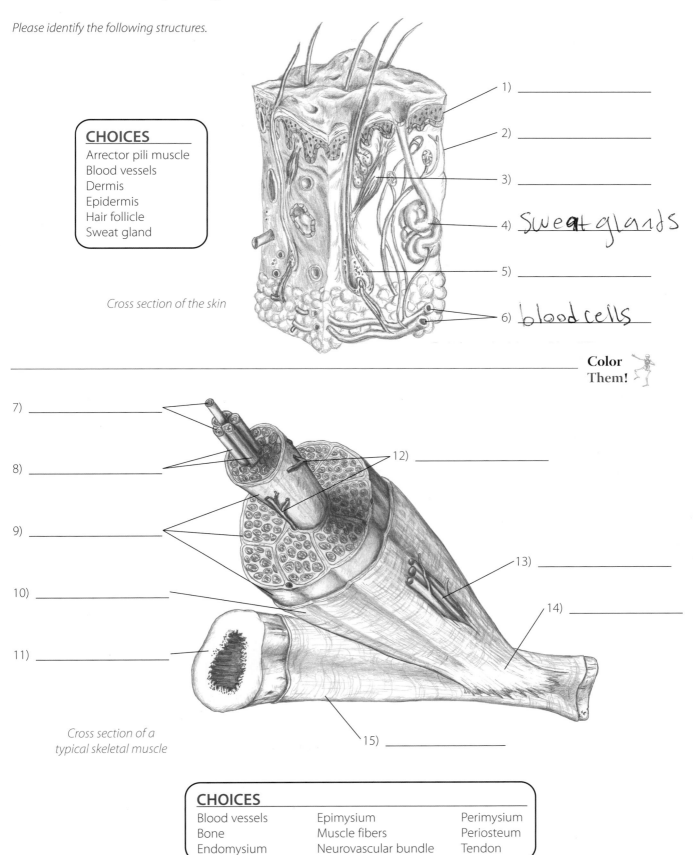

CHOICES
Arrector pili muscle
Blood vessels
Dermis
Epidermis
Hair follicle
Sweat gland

Cross section of the skin

1) _____

2) _____

3) _____

4) sweat glands

5) _____

6) blood cells

Color Them!

7) _____

8) _____

9) _____

10) _____

11) _____

12) _____

13) _____

14) _____

15) _____

Cross section of a typical skeletal muscle

CHOICES

Blood vessels	Epimysium	Perimysium
Bone	Muscle fibers	Periosteum
Endomysium	Neurovascular bundle	Tendon

Please identify the types of muscle bellies and joints.

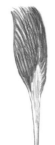
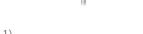
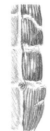
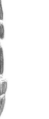

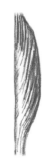

Color Them!

1) _____

2) _____

3) _____

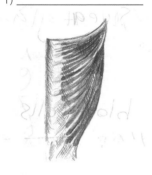
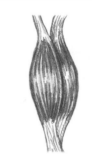
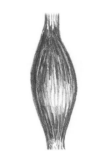

4) _____

5) _____

6) _____

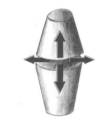
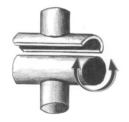
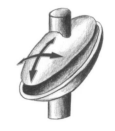

7) _____

8) _____

9) _____

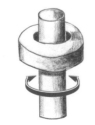
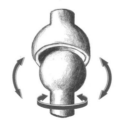
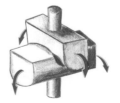

10) _____

11) _____

12) _____

CHOICES

Ball-and-socket	Convergent	Gliding	Pivot
Biceps	Ellipsoid	Hinge	Saddle
Bipennate	Fusiform	Multibelly	Unipennate

Please identify the following structures.

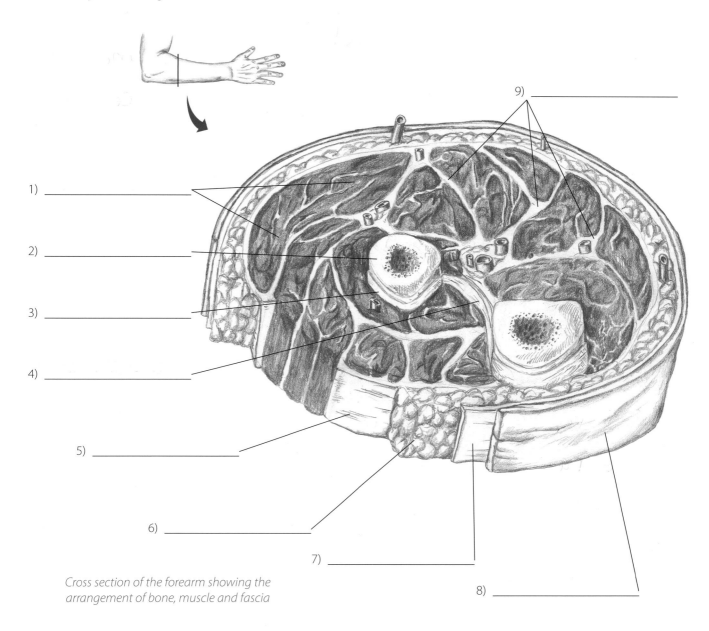

9) _____

1) _____

2) _____

3) _____

4) _____

5) _____

6) _____

7) _____

8) _____

Cross section of the forearm showing the
arrangement of bone, muscle and fascia

Color It!

CHOICES

Adipose (fatty) tissue	Interosseous membrane	Skin
Bone	Muscle tissue	Superficial fascia
Deep fascia (2)	Periosteum	

Please identify the following structures.

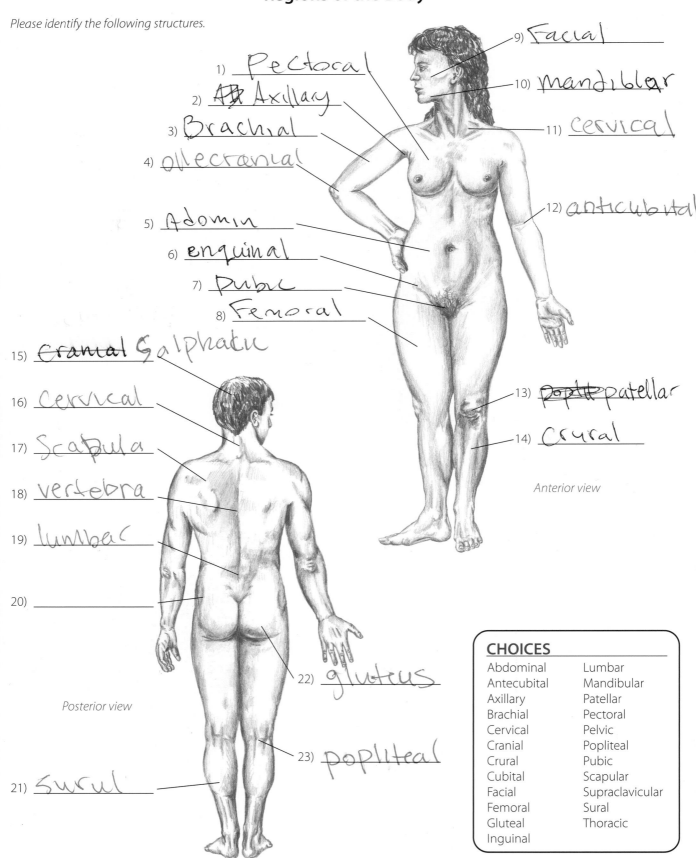

1) Pectoral
2) ~~Ax~~ Axillary
3) Brachial
4) ollecranial
5) Adomin
6) enguinal
7) Pubic
8) Femoral

9) Facial
10) ~~mandiblar~~
11) Cervical
12) anticubital

13) ~~poplit~~ patellar
14) Crural

Anterior view

15) ~~Cranial~~ Salphatic
16) Cervical
17) Scapula
18) vertebra
19) lumbar
20) ____
21) Surul
22) gluteus
23) popliteal

Posterior view

CHOICES

Abdominal	Lumbar
Antecubital	Mandibular
Axillary	Patellar
Brachial	Pectoral
Cervical	Pelvic
Cranial	Popliteal
Crural	Pubic
Cubital	Scapular
Facial	Supraclavicular
Femoral	Sural
Gluteal	Thoracic
Inguinal	

Please identify the following structures.

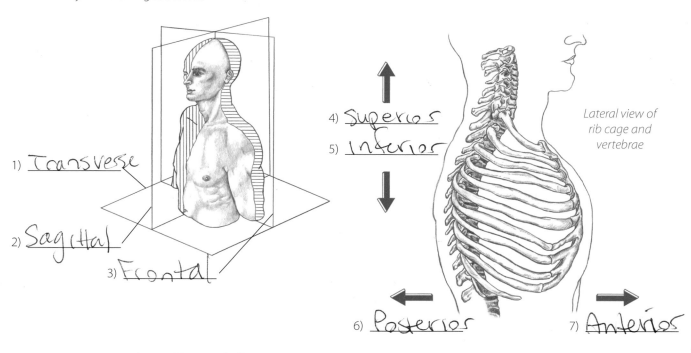

1) _Transverse_

2) _Sagittal_

3) _Frontal_

4) _Superior_

5) _Inferior_

6) _Posterior_

7) _Anterior_

Lateral view of rib cage and vertebrae

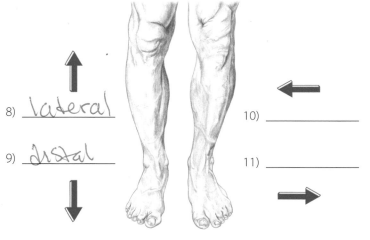

8) _Lateral_

9) _distal_

10) _____

11) _____

Anterior view of legs and feet

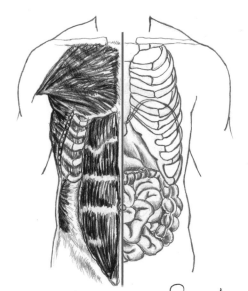

The abdominal muscles are (12) _Superficial_ to the intestines. Likewise, the intestines are (13) _deep_ to the abdominal muscles.

CHOICES

Anterior	Posterior
Deep	Proximal
Distal	Sagittal
Frontal	Superficial
Inferior	Superior
Lateral	Transverse
Medial	

Please match the word to the appropriate definition.

Directions and Positions

1) __c__ anterior
2) __j__ deep
3) __i__ distal
4) __e__ inferior
5) __b__ lateral
6) __h__ medial
7) __a__ posterior
8) __g__ proximal
9) __f__ superficial
10) __d__ superior

a) further toward the back of the body
b) a structure of the arm or leg that is further away from the trunk
c) further toward the front of the body
d) a structure closer to the head
e) a structure closer to the feet
f) a structure closer to the body's surface
g) a structure of the arm or leg that is closer to the trunk
h) closer to the midline of the body
i) further away from the midline of the body
j) a structure deeper in the body

Movements of the Body

11) _____ abduction
12) _____ adduction
13) _____ circumduction
14) _____ dorsiflexion
15) _____ extension
16) _____ flexion
17) _____ lateral flexion
18) _____ lateral rotation
19) _____ medial rotation
20) _____ plantar flexion
21) _____ pronation
22) _____ rotation
23) _____ supination

k) a movement that moves a limb laterally away from the midline
l) a limb at the shoulder or hip turns in toward the midline
m) a limb at the shoulder or hip swings away from the midline
n) a movement bringing the radius and ulna parallel to one another
o) ankle movement stepping on the car's gas pedal
p) a combination of flexion, extension, adduction and abduction
q) when the head or vertebral column bend laterally to the side
r) a movement of the head and vertebral column along the transverse plane
s) a movement that bends a joint or brings the bones closer together
t) ankle movement letting off the car's gas pedal
u) a movement that straightens or opens a joint
v) a movement that brings a limb medially toward the body's midline
w) a movement when the radius crosses over the ulna

Please identify the movement and its location.

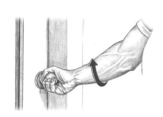

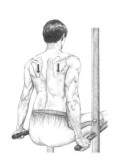

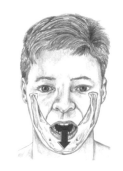

1) <u>supination of the forearm</u>

2) _____

3) _____

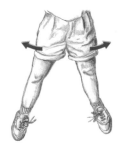

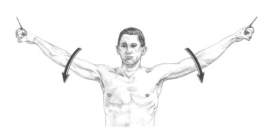

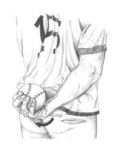

4) _____

5) <u>abduction</u>

6) _____

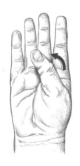

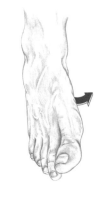

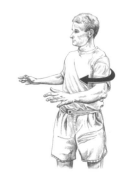

7) _____

8) _____

9) _____

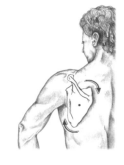

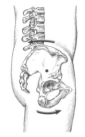

10) _____

11) _____

12) _____

Please identify the movement and its location.

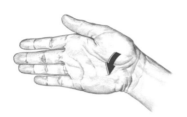

13) _____

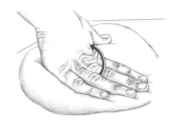

14) _____

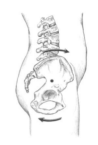

15) _____

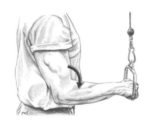

16) _____

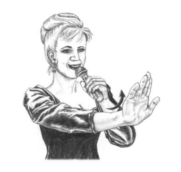

17) _____

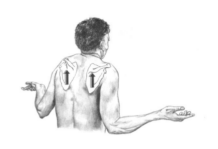

18) _____

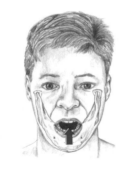

19) _____

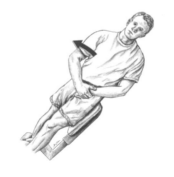

20) _____

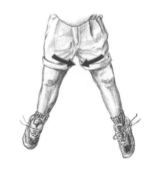

21) _____

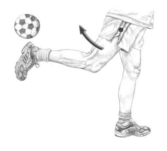

22) _____

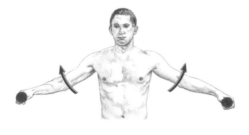

23) _____

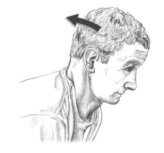

24) _____

Please identify the movement and its location.

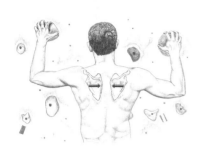

25) _____

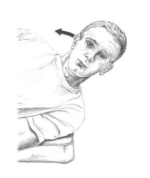

26) _____

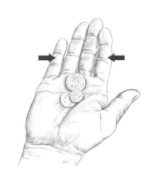

27) _____

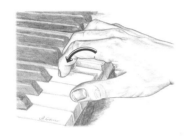

28) _____

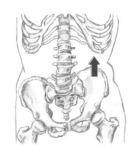

29) _____

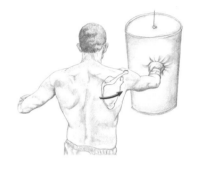

30) _____

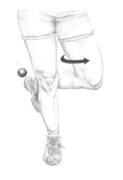

31) _____

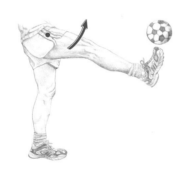

32) _____

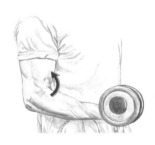

33) _____

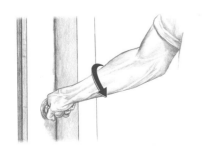

34) _____

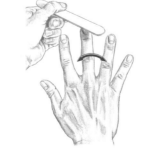

35) _____

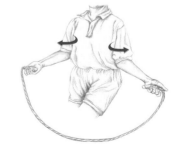

36) _____

Please identify the movement and its location.

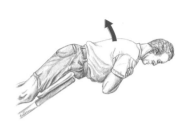
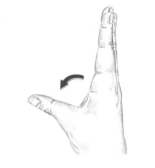
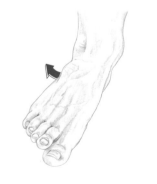

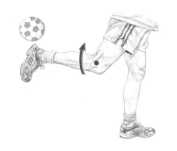
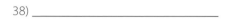
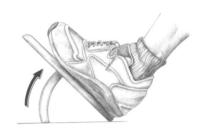
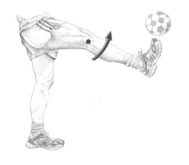
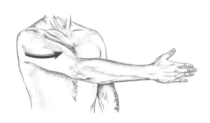
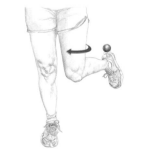

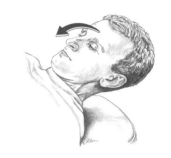
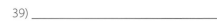
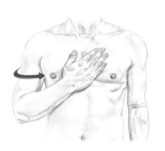
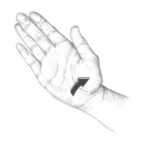
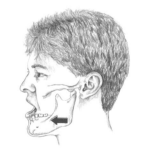

37) _____

38) _____

39) _____

40) _____

41) _____

42) _____

43) _____

44) _____

45) _____

46) _____

47) _____

48) _____

Please identify the movement and its location.

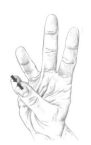

49) _____

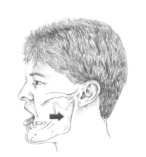

50) _____

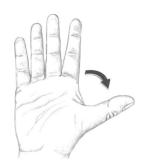

51) _____

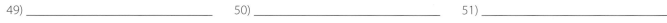

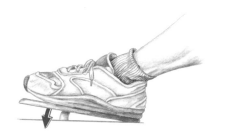

52) _____

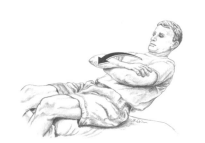

53) _____

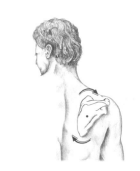

54) _____

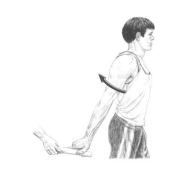

55) _____

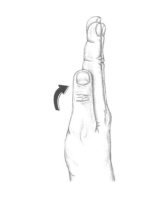

56) _____

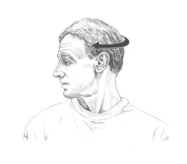

57) _____

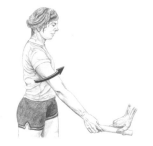

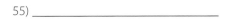

58) _____

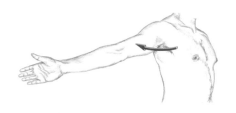

59) _____

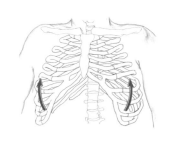

60) _____

Please identify the following structures.

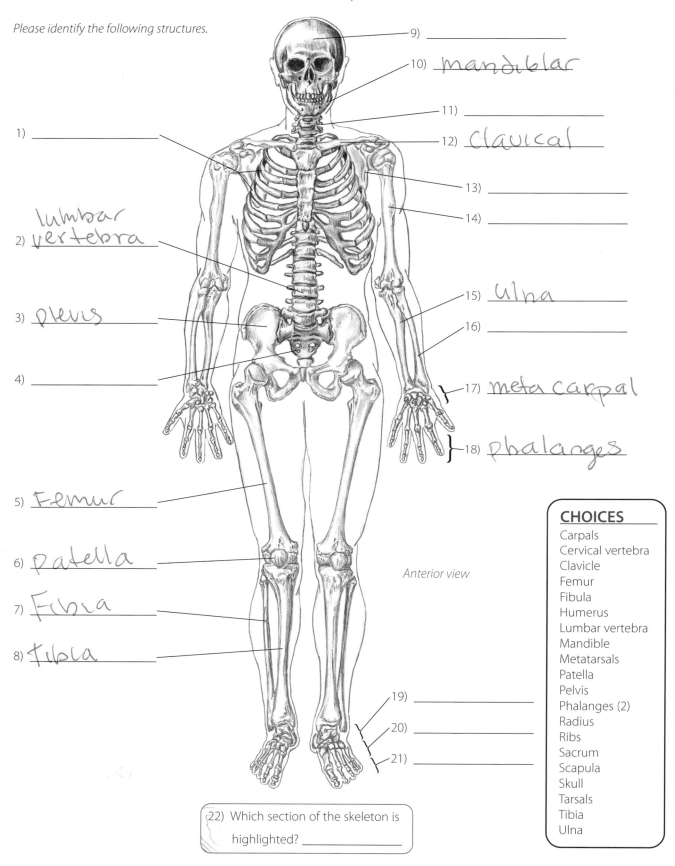

9) _____

10) mandiblar

11) _____

12) clavical

13) _____

14) _____

1) _____

2) lumbar vertebra

15) Ulna

16) _____

3) plevis

4) _____

17) meta carpal

18) phalanges

5) Femur

6) Patella

7) Fibia

8) Tibia

Anterior view

19) _____

20) _____

21) _____

22) Which section of the skeleton is
highlighted? _____

CHOICES
Carpals
Cervical vertebra
Clavicle
Femur
Fibula
Humerus
Lumbar vertebra
Mandible
Metatarsals
Patella
Pelvis
Phalanges (2)
Radius
Ribs
Sacrum
Scapula
Skull
Tarsals
Tibia
Ulna

Please identify the following structures.

1) _____

2) _____

3) _____

4) _____

5) _____

6) _____

7) _____

8) _____

9) _____

10) _____

11) _____

12) _____

13) _____

14) _____

Posterior view

15) _____

16) _____

17) _____

18) _____

19) _____

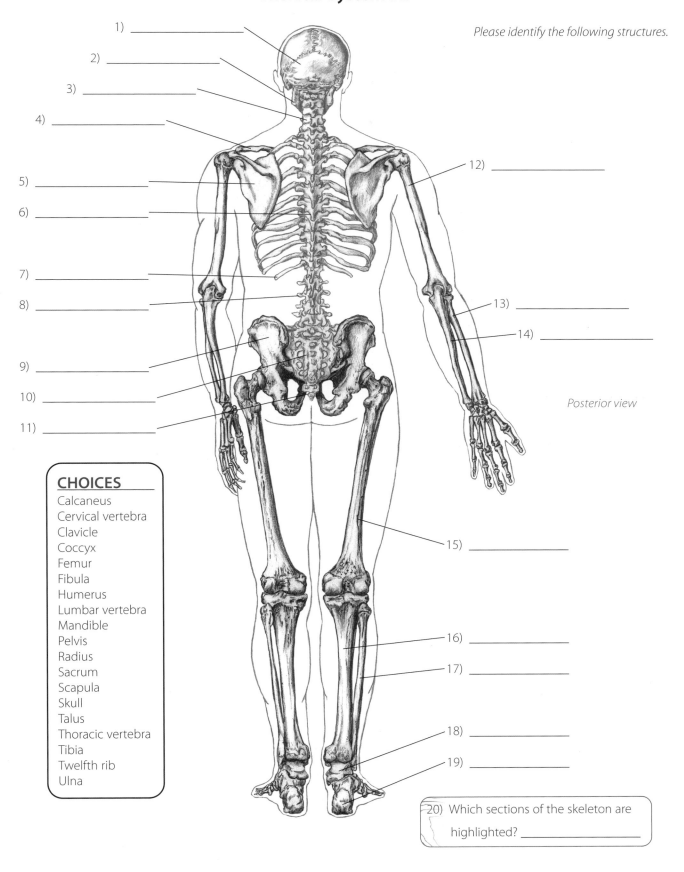

CHOICES

Calcaneus
Cervical vertebra
Clavicle
Coccyx
Femur
Fibula
Humerus
Lumbar vertebra
Mandible
Pelvis
Radius
Sacrum
Scapula
Skull
Talus
Thoracic vertebra
Tibia
Twelfth rib
Ulna

20) Which sections of the skeleton are

highlighted? _____

Please identify the following structures.

1) _____

2) _____

3) *deltoid*

4) _____

5) *biceps bracial*

6) _____

7) _____

8) _____

9) *Abdominal*

10) _____

11) _____

12) _____

13) _____

14) _____

15) _____

16) _____

17) _____

18) _____

19) _____

20) _____

21) _____

22) _____

23) _____

24) _____

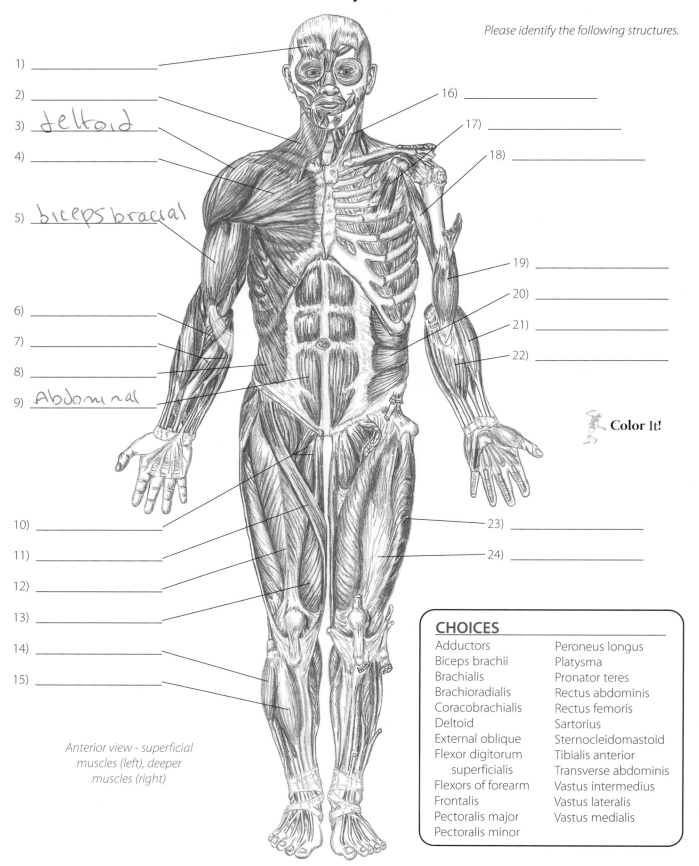

Color It!

Anterior view - superficial muscles (left), deeper muscles (right)

CHOICES

Adductors	Peroneus longus
Biceps brachii	Platysma
Brachialis	Pronator teres
Brachioradialis	Rectus abdominis
Coracobrachialis	Rectus femoris
Deltoid	Sartorius
External oblique	Sternocleidomastoid
Flexor digitorum	Tibialis anterior
superficialis	Transverse abdominis
Flexors of forearm	Vastus intermedius
Frontalis	Vastus lateralis
Pectoralis major	Vastus medialis
Pectoralis minor	

16

Please identify the following structures.

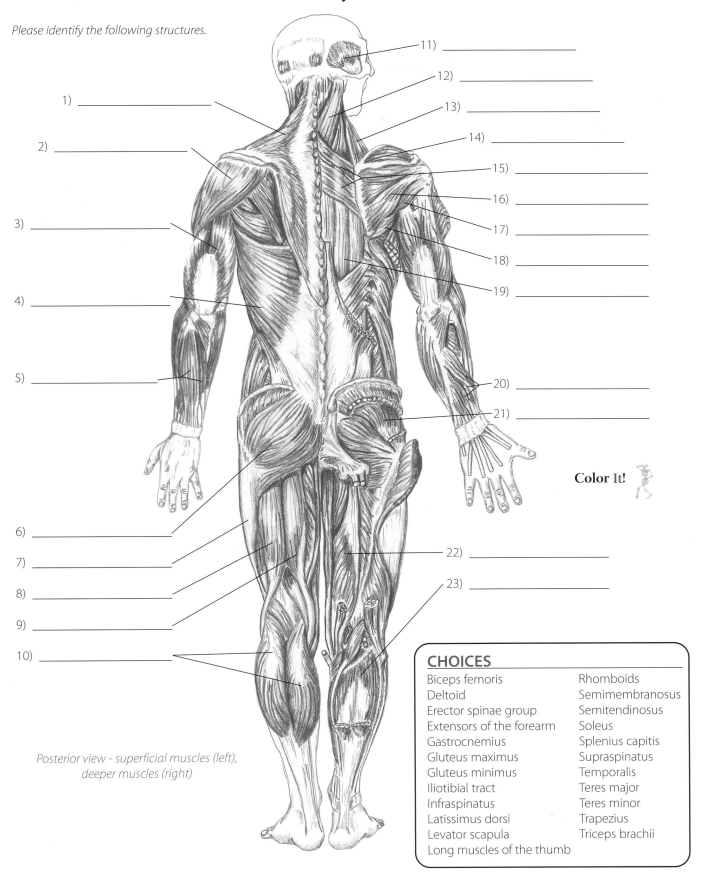

1) _____

2) _____

3) _____

4) _____

5) _____

6) _____

7) _____

8) _____

9) _____

10) _____

11) _____

12) _____

13) _____

14) _____

15) _____

16) _____

17) _____

18) _____

19) _____

20) _____

21) _____

22) _____

23) _____

Color It!

*Posterior view - superficial muscles (left),
deeper muscles (right)*

CHOICES

Biceps femoris	Rhomboids
Deltoid	Semimembranosus
Erector spinae group	Semitendinosus
Extensors of the forearm	Soleus
Gastrocnemius	Splenius capitis
Gluteus maximus	Supraspinatus
Gluteus minimus	Temporalis
Iliotibial tract	Teres major
Infraspinatus	Teres minor
Latissimus dorsi	Trapezius
Levator scapula	Triceps brachii
Long muscles of the thumb	

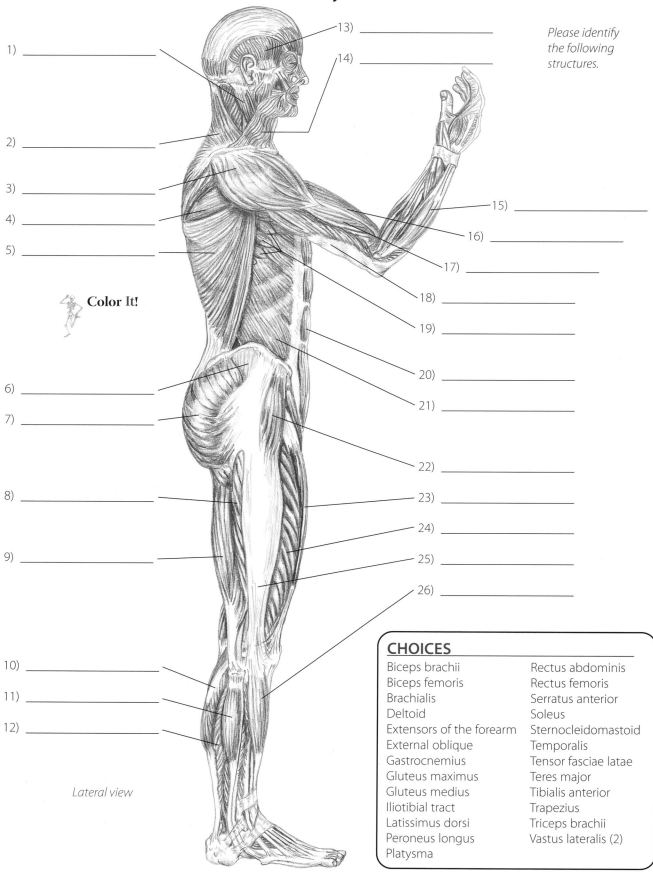

13) _____

14) _____

Please identify the following structures.

1) _____

2) _____

3) _____

4) _____

5) _____

Color It!

6) _____

7) _____

8) _____

9) _____

10) _____

11) _____

12) _____

15) _____

16) _____

17) _____

18) _____

19) _____

20) _____

21) _____

22) _____

23) _____

24) _____

25) _____

26) _____

Lateral view

CHOICES

Biceps brachii	Rectus abdominis
Biceps femoris	Rectus femoris
Brachialis	Serratus anterior
Deltoid	Soleus
Extensors of the forearm	Sternocleidomastoid
External oblique	Temporalis
Gastrocnemius	Tensor fasciae latae
Gluteus maximus	Teres major
Gluteus medius	Tibialis anterior
Iliotibial tract	Trapezius
Latissimus dorsi	Triceps brachii
Peroneus longus	Vastus lateralis (2)
Platysma	

18

Please identify the following structures.

CHOICES

Antebrachial fascia
Biceps brachii
Brachial fascia
Extensor muscles
Flexor muscles
Humerus
Interosseous membrane
Lateral intermuscular septum
Medial intermuscular septum
Radius
Triceps brachii
Ulna

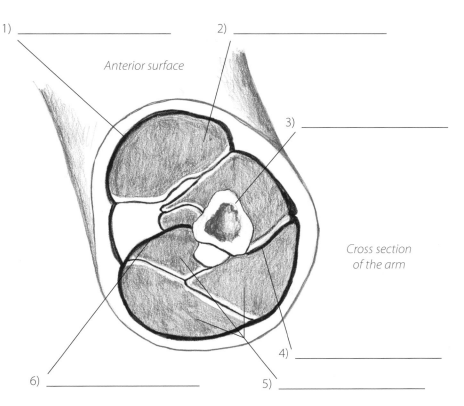

1) _____

2) _____

3) _____

4) _____

5) _____

6) _____

Anterior surface

Cross section of the arm

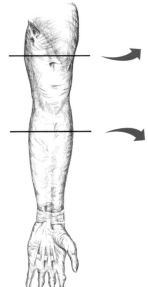

Anterior view of the left arm and forearm, skin removed

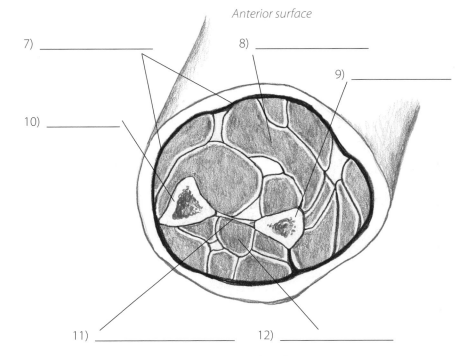

Anterior surface

7) _____

8) _____

9) _____

10) _____

11) _____

12) _____

Cross section of the forearm

Please identify the following structures.

1) _____

2) _____

3) _____

Cross section of the thigh

4) _____

5) _____

6) _____

7) _____

8) _____

Posterior surface

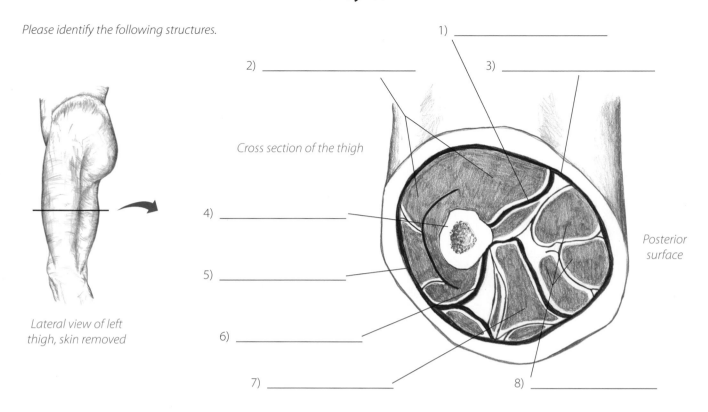

Lateral view of left thigh, skin removed

9) _____

10) _____

Anterior surface

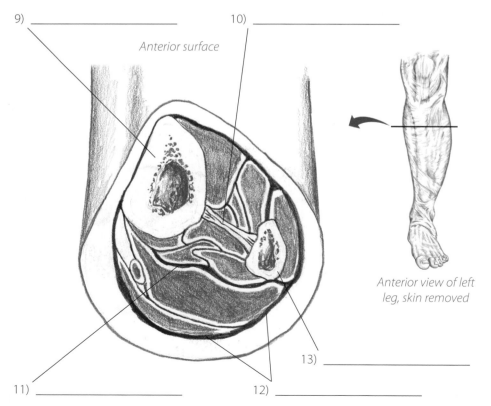

11) _____

12) _____

13) _____

Cross section of the leg

Anterior view of left leg, skin removed

CHOICES

Adductors
Crural fascia
Deep crural fascia
Fascia lata
Femur
Fibula
Hamstrings
Iliotibial tract
Interosseous membrane
Lateral intermuscular septum
Medial intermuscular septum
Quadriceps
Tibia

Please identify the following structures.

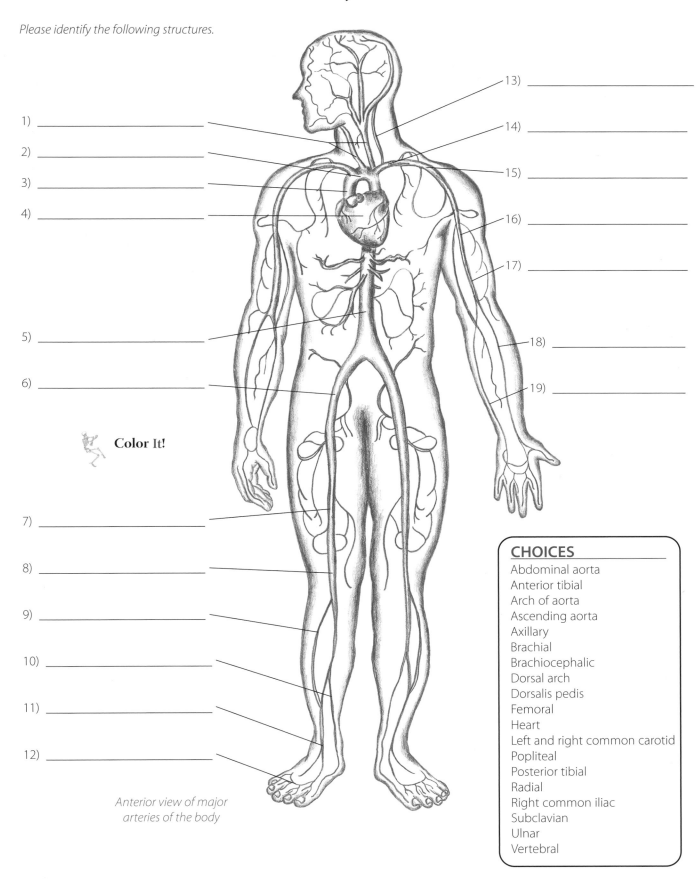

1) _____

2) _____

3) _____

4) _____

5) _____

6) _____

Color It!

7) _____

8) _____

9) _____

10) _____

11) _____

12) _____

13) _____

14) _____

15) _____

16) _____

17) _____

18) _____

19) _____

*Anterior view of major
arteries of the body*

CHOICES
Abdominal aorta
Anterior tibial
Arch of aorta
Ascending aorta
Axillary
Brachial
Brachiocephalic
Dorsal arch
Dorsalis pedis
Femoral
Heart
Left and right common carotid
Popliteal
Posterior tibial
Radial
Right common iliac
Subclavian
Ulnar
Vertebral

Please identify the following structures.

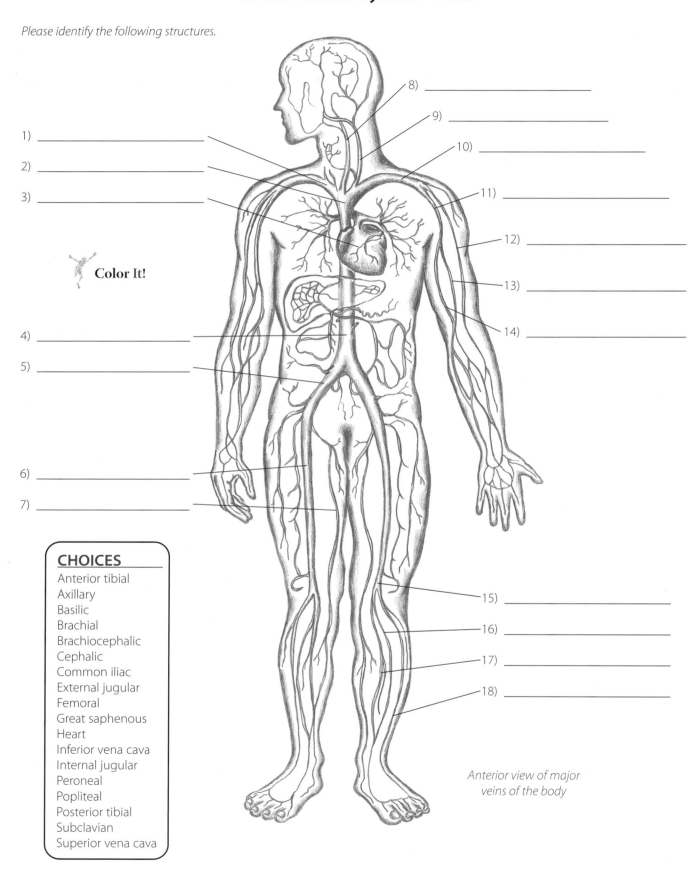

8) _____

9) _____

1) _____

10) _____

2) _____

11) _____

3) _____

12) _____

Color It!

13) _____

14) _____

4) _____

5) _____

6) _____

7) _____

CHOICES
Anterior tibial
Axillary
Basilic
Brachial
Brachiocephalic
Cephalic
Common iliac
External jugular
Femoral
Great saphenous
Heart
Inferior vena cava
Internal jugular
Peroneal
Popliteal
Posterior tibial
Subclavian
Superior vena cava

15) _____

16) _____

17) _____

18) _____

*Anterior view of major
veins of the body*

22

Please identify the following structures.

1) _____

2) _____

3) _____

4) _____

5) _____

6) _____

7) _____

8) _____

9) _____

10) _____

11) _____

12) _____

13) _____

14) _____

15) _____

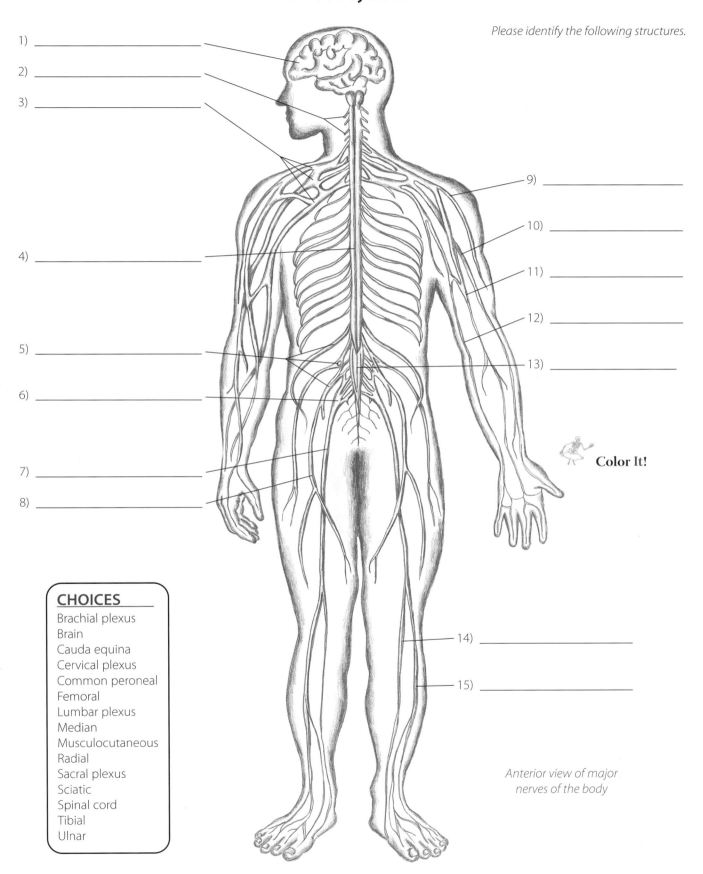

Color It!

CHOICES

Brachial plexus
Brain
Cauda equina
Cervical plexus
Common peroneal
Femoral
Lumbar plexus
Median
Musculocutaneous
Radial
Sacral plexus
Sciatic
Spinal cord
Tibial
Ulnar

Anterior view of major nerves of the body

Please identify the following structures.

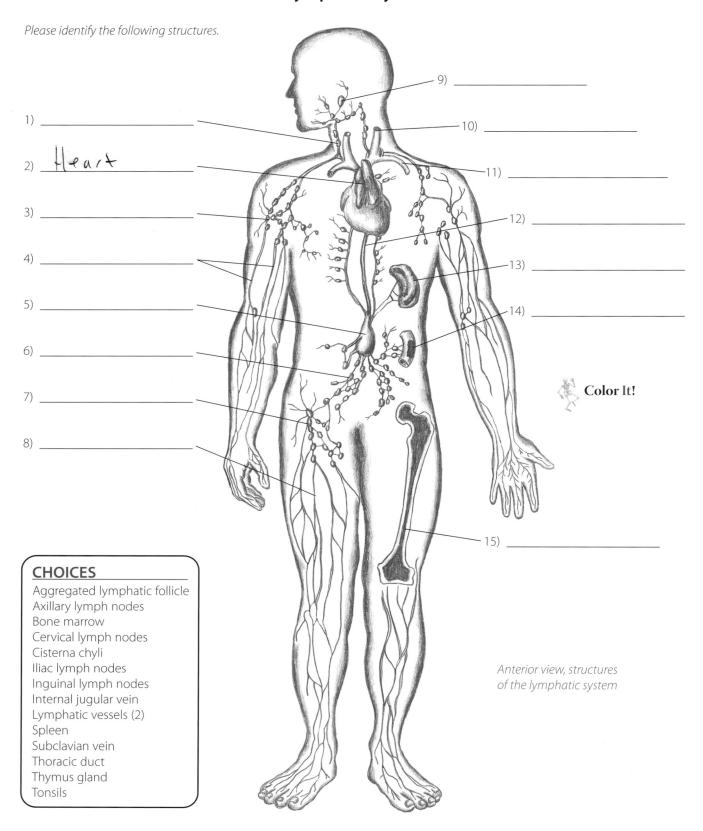

1) _____

2) *Heart* _____

3) _____

4) _____

5) _____

6) _____

7) _____

8) _____

9) _____

10) _____

11) _____

12) _____

13) _____

14) _____

15) _____

Color It!

Anterior view, structures of the lymphatic system

CHOICES
Aggregated lymphatic follicle
Axillary lymph nodes
Bone marrow
Cervical lymph nodes
Cisterna chyli
Iliac lymph nodes
Inguinal lymph nodes
Internal jugular vein
Lymphatic vessels (2)
Spleen
Subclavian vein
Thoracic duct
Thymus gland
Tonsils

24

Please identify the following structures.

CHOICES

Acromion
Axilla
Biceps brachii
Clavicle
Deltoid (2)
Inferior angle of the scapula
Latissimus dorsi (2)
Pectoralis major
Serratus anterior
Spine of the scapula
Superior nuchal line of the occiput
Trapezius (2)
Triceps brachii (2)

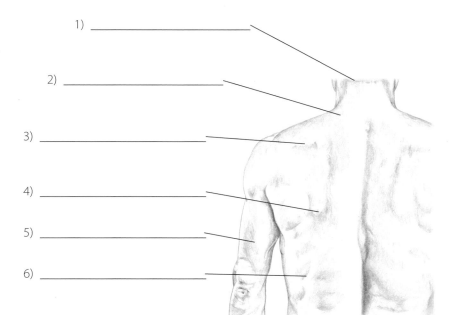

1) _____

2) _____

3) _____

4) _____

5) _____

6) _____

Posterior view

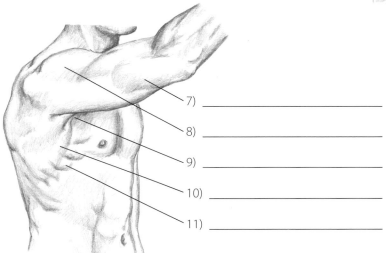

7) _____

8) _____

9) _____

10) _____

11) _____

Anterior/lateral view

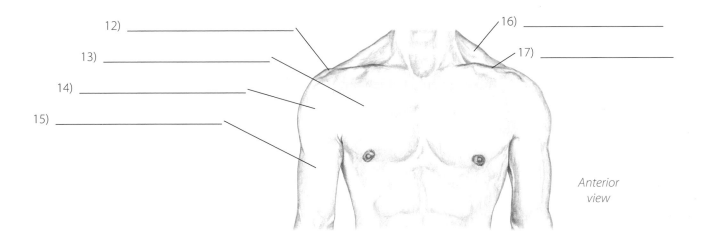

12) _____

13) _____

14) _____

15) _____

16) _____

17) _____

Anterior view

Please answer the following questions.

1) Three bones that make up the shoulder complex are the _____, _____ and

_____.

2) The acromioclavicular and sternoclavicular are what types of joints? _____

3) The single attachment between the axial and upper appendicular skeletons is the _____ joint.

4) The humerus and scapula form the _____ joint.

5) A great base camp for locating other bony landmarks of the shoulder is the _____.

6) With your partner prone, how can you best position your partner's hand to locate the inferior angle of the scapula?

_____

7) A "winged scapula" often indicates weakness in which muscle? _____

8) The superior angle of the scapula serves as an attachment site for the _____ muscle

and is deep to the _____ muscle.

9) When accessing the lateral border of the scapula, through which two muscle bellies will you have to palpate?

_____   _____

10) Accessing the infraglenoid tubercle can elicit tenderness. How can you palpate this landmark without causing pain?

_____

Let's Palpate!

Remember - there are no right or wrong answers here

Locate and explore the **coracoid process of the scapula** on three individuals. Then write three words that describe what you feel. (See p. 67 in *Trail Guide*)

Person #1 _____   Person #2 _____   Person #3 _____

_____   _____   _____

_____   _____   _____

_____   _____   _____

Please answer the following questions.

1) The three scapular fossae contain which three muscles?

_____ _____ _____

2) The infraspinous fossa can be isolated by setting your fingers on which three bony landmarks?

_____ _____ _____

3) Palpating laterally along the supraspinous fossa, your fingers will bump into which two bony structures?

_____ _____

4) To locate the subscapular fossa in a sidelying position, you slowly sink your thumb onto the fossa's surface. What can your

other hand do to help access the fossa? _____

5) To access the medial portion of the subscapular fossa, how would you position your partner?

_____

6) The acromion serves as an attachment site for which two muscles?

_____ _____

7) When palpating the clavicle, the _____ end rises superiorly while the _____
end curves inferiorly.

8) To feel the acromioclavicular joint space widen slightly and then diminish, you can ask your partner to do

which two movements of the scapula? _____ _____

9) The coracoid process is often located in the _____ groove.

10) Sculpting a circle around the edges of the coracoid process can help you get a better understanding of its

_____ and _____.

11) What are the three muscles that attach to the greater tubercle of the humerus?

_____ _____ _____

12) Within the intertubercular groove lies the tendon of which muscle? _____

Extra Credit

How many muscles attach to the scapula? _____ Try listing them below.

1) _____

*Please identify the following structures. Numbers in **bold** indicate bones.*

2) _____

3) _____

4) _____

5) _____

6) _____

Color It!

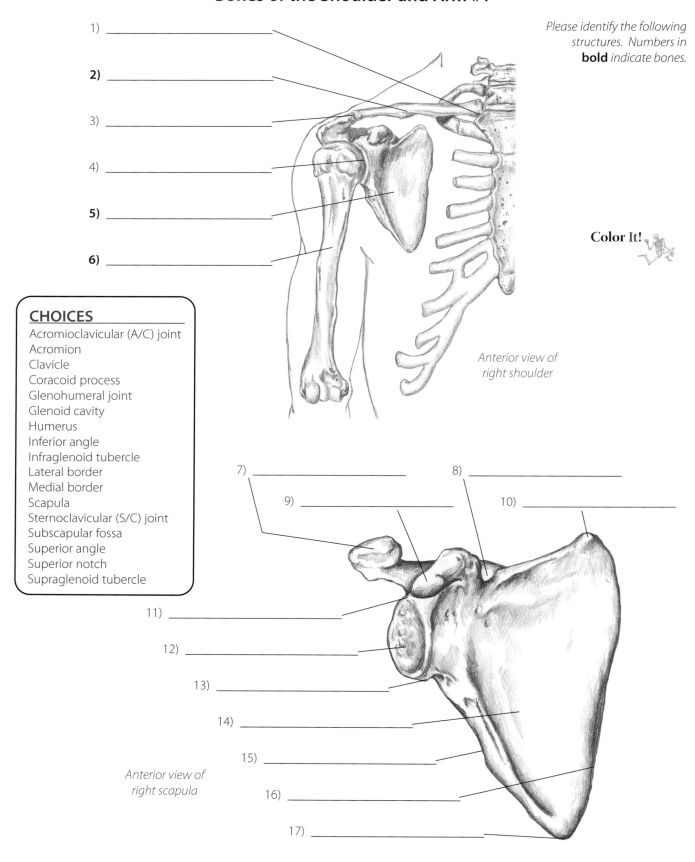

Anterior view of right shoulder

CHOICES
Acromioclavicular (A/C) joint
Acromion
Clavicle
Coracoid process
Glenohumeral joint
Glenoid cavity
Humerus
Inferior angle
Infraglenoid tubercle
Lateral border
Medial border
Scapula
Sternoclavicular (S/C) joint
Subscapular fossa
Superior angle
Superior notch
Supraglenoid tubercle

7) _____

8) _____

9) _____

10) _____

11) _____

12) _____

13) _____

14) _____

15) _____

Anterior view of right scapula

16) _____

17) _____

Please identify the following structures.

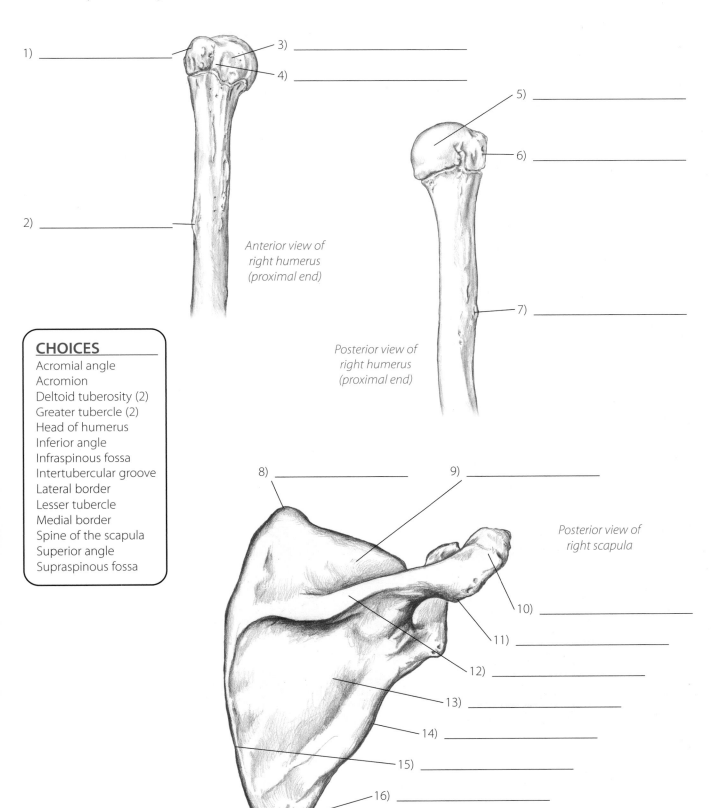

1) _____

2) _____

3) _____

4) _____

5) _____

6) _____

7) _____

Anterior view of right humerus (proximal end)

Posterior view of right humerus (proximal end)

CHOICES
Acromial angle
Acromion
Deltoid tuberosity (2)
Greater tubercle (2)
Head of humerus
Inferior angle
Infraspinous fossa
Intertubercular groove
Lateral border
Lesser tubercle
Medial border
Spine of the scapula
Superior angle
Supraspinous fossa

8) _____

9) _____

Posterior view of right scapula

10) _____

11) _____

12) _____

13) _____

14) _____

15) _____

16) _____

Please identify the following structures.

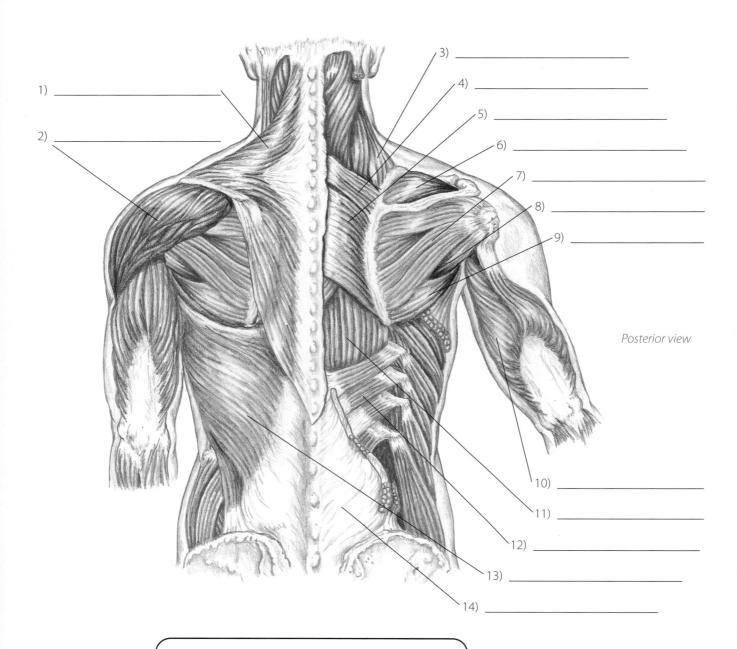

Posterior view

1) _____
2) _____
3) _____
4) _____
5) _____
6) _____
7) _____
8) _____
9) _____
10) _____
11) _____
12) _____
13) _____
14) _____

CHOICES

Deltoid	Serratus posterior inferior
Erector spinae group	Supraspinatus
Infraspinatus	Teres major
Latissimus dorsi	Teres minor
Levator scapula	Thoracolumbar aponeurosis
Rhomboid major	Trapezius
Rhomboid minor	Triceps brachii

Please identify the following structures.

CHOICES

Biceps brachii (2)   Pectoralis major
Brachialis   Pectoralis minor
Coracobrachialis   Serratus anterior (2)
Deltoid (2)   Teres major
External oblique   Teres minor
Infraspinatus   Trapezius (2)
Latissimus dorsi (2) Triceps brachii
Levator scapula

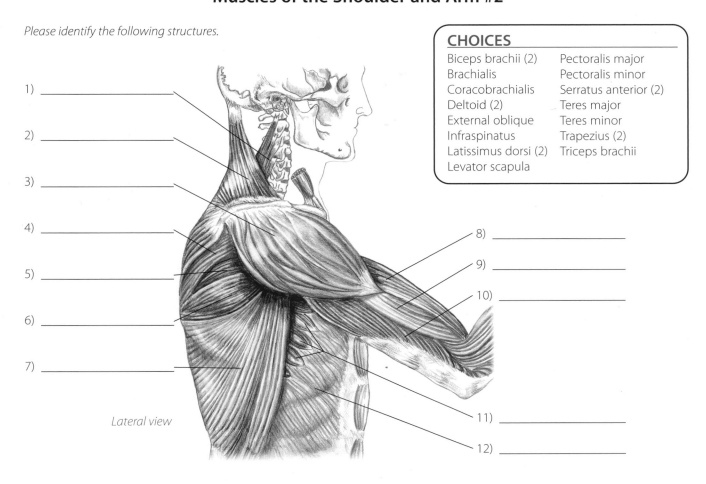

1) _____

2) _____

3) _____

4) _____

5) _____

6) _____

7) _____

Lateral view

8) _____

9) _____

10) _____

11) _____

12) _____

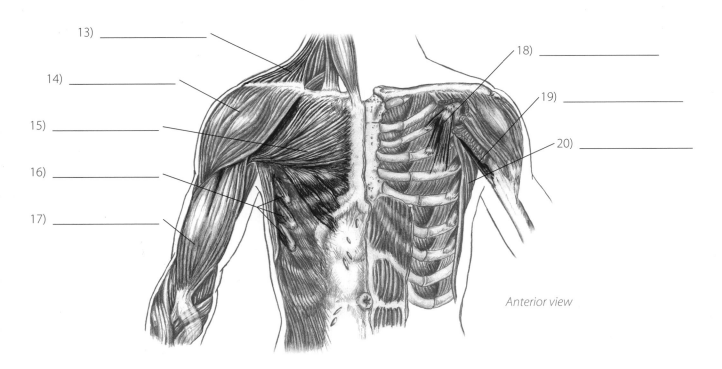

13) _____

14) _____

15) _____

16) _____

17) _____

18) _____

19) _____

20) _____

Anterior view

Using different colors, please fill in and label the muscles and other structures listed below.

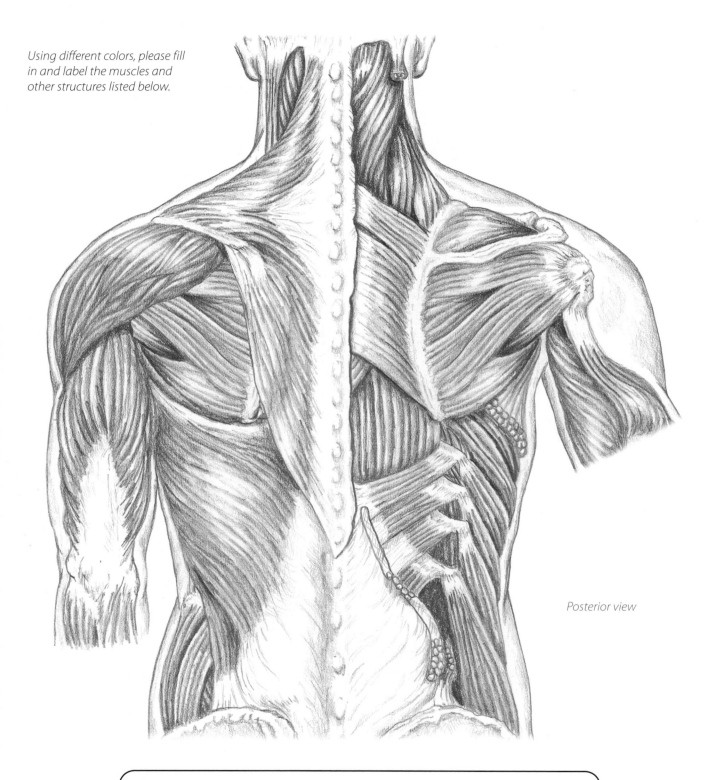

Posterior view

Deltoid	Rhomboid major	Teres minor
Erector spinae group	Rhomboid minor	Thoracolumbar aponeurosis
Infraspinatus	Serratus posterior inferior	Trapezius
Latissimus dorsi	Supraspinatus	Triceps brachii
Levator scapula	Teres major	

Using different colors, please fill in and label the muscles listed below.

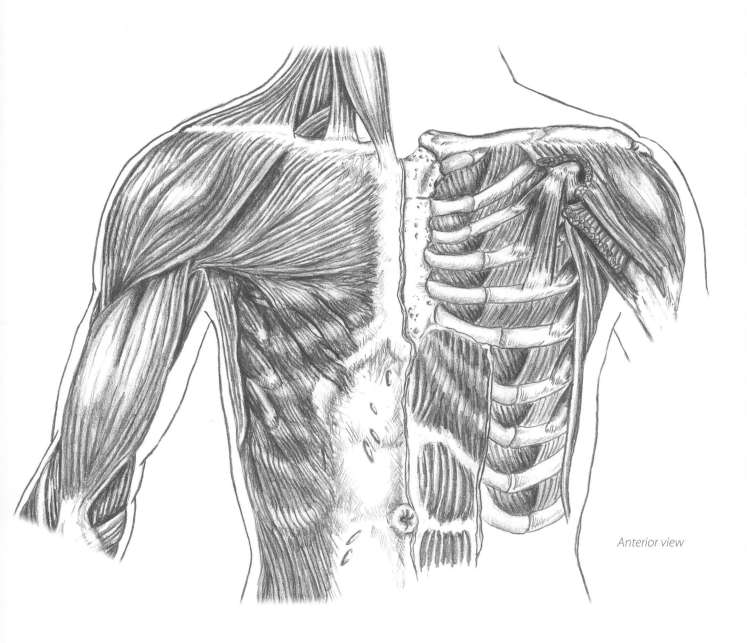

Anterior view

Biceps brachii   Pectoralis major   Serratus anterior
Coracobrachialis   Pectoralis minor   Sternocleidomastoid
Deltoid   Rectus abdominis   Trapezius
Latissimus dorsi

Please list the action demonstrated, two synergists and one antagonist.
The first letter of the muscles has been provided.

1) This action happens at which joint?

_____

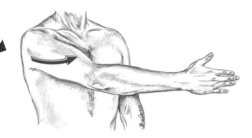

2) Action

_____

3) Synergists

D _____

P _____

4) Antagonist

I _____

5) Action

_____

6) Synergists

T _____

R _____

7) Antagonist

P _____

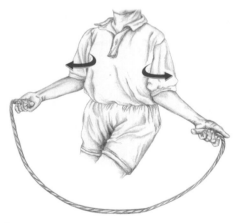

8) Action

_____

9) Synergists

D _____

T _____

10) Antagonist

S _____

Please list the action demonstrated, two synergists and one antagonist.
The first letter of the muscles has been provided.

1) This action happens at which joint?

_____

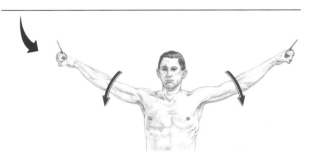

2) Action

_____

3) Synergists

I _____

T _____

4) Antagonist

S _____

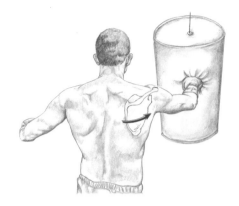

8) Action

_____

9) Synergists

S _____

P _____

10) Antagonist

R _____

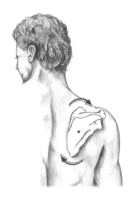

5) Action

_____

6) Synergists

R _____

L _____

7) Antagonist

T _____

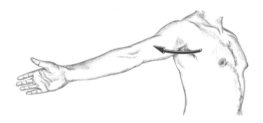

11) Action

_____

12) Synergists

I _____

T _____

13) Antagonist

P _____

Please list the action demonstrated, two synergists and one antagonist.
The first letter of the muscles has been provided.

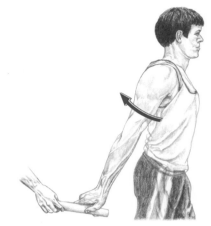

1) This action happens at which joint?

_____

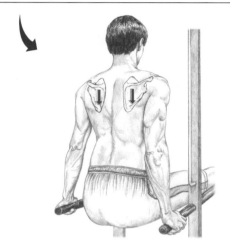

2) Action

_____

3) Synergists

S _____

P _____

4) Antagonist

R _____

5) Action

_____

6) Synergists

D _____

L _____

7) Antagonist

B _____

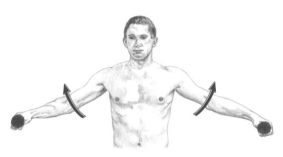

8) Action

_____

9) Synergists

D _____

S _____

10) Antagonist

P _____

Please list the action demonstrated, synergist(s) and antagonist(s).
The first letter of the muscles has been provided.

1) This action happens at which joint?

_____

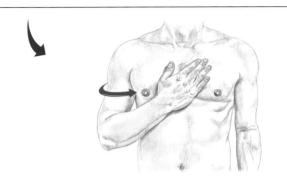

2) Action

_____

3) Synergists

S _____

P _____

4) Antagonist

I _____

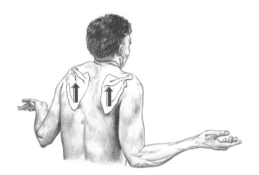

5) Action

_____

6) Synergists

R _____

L _____

7) Antagonist

S _____

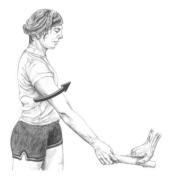

8) Action

_____

9) Synergists

B _____

C _____

10) Antagonist

L _____

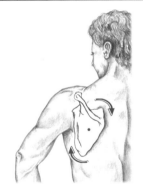

11) Action

_____

12) Synergist

T _____

13) Antagonists

R _____

R _____

Please identify the following muscles.

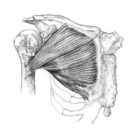

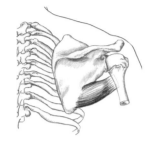

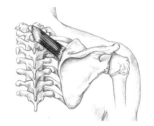

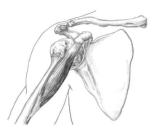

1) _____

2) _____

3) _____

4) _____

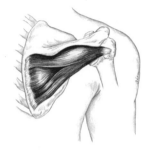

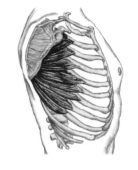

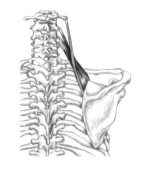

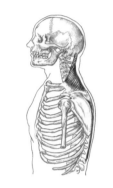

5) _____

6) _____

7) _____

8) _____

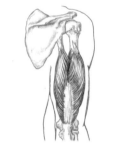

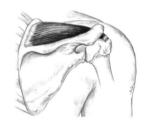

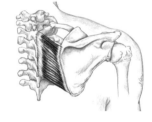

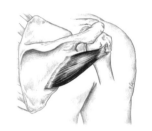

9) _____

10) _____

11) _____

12) _____

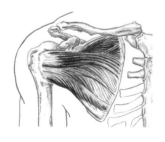

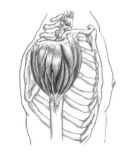

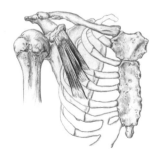

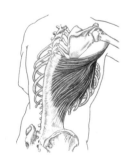

13) _____

14) _____

15) _____

16) _____

Please answer the following questions.

1) The *origin* of the deltoid is identical to the *insertion* of which muscle? _____

2) What action can you ask your client to perform in order to contract all fibers of the deltoid?

   _____

3) The actions of the deltoid's anterior and posterior fibers make it an _____ to itself.

4) The upper fibers of the trapezius elevate the scapula, so the lower fibers must

   _____ the scapula.

5) Bilateral contraction of the upper fibers of the trapezius will create what movement of the head and neck?

   _____

6) To feel the middle fibers of the trapezius contract, you could ask your partner to perform which action?

   _____

7) Which portion of the latissimus dorsi is easy to grasp? _____

8) When palpating the latissimus dorsi, how can you discern the muscle tissue from the superficial skin?

   _____

9) One palpatory distinction between the teres major and latissimus dorsi is that the teres attaches to the

   _____ of the scapula.

Shorten or Lengthen?

10) Passive abduction of the scapula would _____ the middle fibers of the trapezius.

11) Passive elevation of the scapula would _____ the trapezius' upper fibers and _____ its lower fibers.

12) Passive rotation of the head and neck to the left would _____ the left trapezius' upper fibers.

13) Passive flexion of the shoulder would _____ the anterior fibers of the deltoid.

14) Passive lateral rotation of the shoulder would _____ the deltoid's posterior fibers.

15) Passive flexion of the shoulder would _____ the latissimus dorsi.

16) Passive adduction of the shoulder would _____ the teres major.

17) Passive medial rotation of the shoulder would _____ the latissimus dorsi and teres major.

Matching

Match the origin and insertion to the correct muscle.

Origins

1) External occipital protuberance, medial portion of superior nuchal line of the occiput, ligamentum nuchae and spinous processes of C-7 through T-12

2) Lateral one-third of clavicle, acromion and spine of the scapula

3) Lateral side of inferior angle and lower half of lateral border of scapula

4) Spinous processes of last six thoracic vertebrae, last three or four ribs, thoracolumbar aponeurosis and posterior iliac crest

Insertions

5) Crest of the lesser tubercle of the humerus (2)

6) Deltoid tuberosity

7) Lateral one-third of clavicle, acromion and spine of the scapula

Muscle	O	I
Deltoid	_____	_____
Latissimus dorsi	_____	_____
Teres major	_____	_____
Trapezius	_____	_____

Let's Palpate!

Remember - there are no right or wrong answers here

Locate and explore the **upper fibers of the trapezius** on three individuals. Then write three words that describe what you feel. (See p. 76-77 in *Trail Guide*)

Person #1 _____   Person #2 _____   Person #3 _____

_____   _____   _____

_____   _____   _____

_____   _____   _____

Please answer the following questions.

1) The four rotator cuff muscles encompass and stabilize the _____ joint.

2) To locate the supraspinatus belly, you must palpate through which muscle? _____

3) The only rotator cuff muscle not involved with rotation of the shoulder is the _____.

4) The dense quality of the infraspinatus is due to its _____.

5) The subscapularis is sandwiched between which fossa and which muscle?

_____   _____

6) What is the best action to ask your partner to perform to feel the supraspinatus contract?

_____

7) What three bony landmarks can you lay your fingers along to isolate the belly of the infraspinatus?

_____   _____   _____

8) If you follow the fibers of the infraspinatus laterally, they converge underneath which muscle?

_____

9) You can distinguish the teres minor from the teres major by their sizes and actions. Explain.

_____

10) When accessing the subscapularis from a sidelying position, under what two muscles should you slide your thumb?

_____   _____

11) What action could you ask your partner to do to gently contract the subscapularis?

_____

12) To access the supraspinatus tendon, you need to sink your thumb tip through which muscle? _____

13) To locate the infraspinatus and teres minor tendons in a supine position, how would you position your partner's shoulder?

_____

14) The subscapularis tendon can be located between the two tendons of which muscle? _____

15) In which two directions do you want to move from the coracoid process to locate the subscapularis tendon?

_____   _____

Matching

Match the origin and insertion to the correct muscle.

Origins

1) Infraspinous fossa of the scapula

2) Subscapular fossa of the scapula

3) Superior half of lateral border of the scapula

4) Supraspinous fossa of the scapula

Muscle	O	I
Infraspinatus	_____	_____
Subscapularis	_____	_____
Supraspinatus	_____	_____
Teres minor	_____	_____

Insertions

5) Greater tubercle of the humerus (3)

6) Lesser tubercle of the humerus

Shorten or Lengthen?

7) Passive medial rotation of the shoulder would _____ the infraspinatus.

8) Passive abduction of the shoulder would _____ the supraspinatus.

9) Passive flexion of the shoulder would _____ the teres minor.

10) Passive lateral rotation of the shoulder would _____ the subscapularis.

Let's Palpate!

Remember - there are no right or wrong answers here

Locate and explore the **infraspinatus** on three individuals. Then write three words that describe what you feel.
(See p. 85 in *Trail Guide*)

Person #1 _____

Person #2 _____

Person #3 _____

_____

_____

_____

_____

_____

_____

_____

_____

_____

Please answer the following questions.

1) The rhomboids are deep to the _____ muscle and superficial to the _____ muscles.

2) Can you name two actions in which the rhomboids and trapezius are synergists and one action in which they are

   antagonists? _____ _____ _____

3) The levator scapula is situated between which two muscles on the lateral side of the neck?

   _____ _____

4) An action to ask your partner to perform to feel the levator scapula contract is _____.

5) When accessing the levator scapula in a supine position, the benefits of rotating the head 45° away from the
   side you are palpating include:

   _____ _____ _____

6) The serratus anterior abducts the scapula, making it a direct antagonist to the _____.

7) Most of the serratus anterior is deep to the scapula and which two muscles?

   _____ _____

8) Accessing the medial portion of the serratus anterior by curling your fingers around the medial border of the
   scapula, your fingers will inherently have to work through the bellies of which two muscles?

   _____ _____

9) The pectoralis major is divided into three segments:

   _____ _____ _____

10) Can you name an everday action in which you use your pectoralis major? _____

11) The most important aspect when palpating near breast tissue is:

   _____

12) If you follow the fibers of the pectoralis major laterally, they blend with the fibers of which muscle?

   _____

13) Flexing the shoulder and pulling it anteriorly while you palpate the pectoralis major in a sidelying position has
    which two benefits?

   _____ _____

14) The pectoralis minor has the potential to create neurovascular compression on which three vessels?

   _____ _____ _____

Matching

Match the origin and insertion to the correct muscle.

Origins

1) First rib and cartilage

2) Medial half of clavicle, sternum and cartilage of first through sixth ribs

3) Spinous processes of C-7 and T-1

4) Spinous processes of T-2 to T-5

5) Surfaces of upper eight or nine ribs

6) Third, fourth and fifth ribs

7) Transverse processes of first through fourth cervical vertebrae

Insertions

8) Anterior surface of medial border of the scapula

9) Coracoid process of the scapula

10) Crest of greater tubercle of the humerus

11) Inferior, lateral aspect of clavicle

12) Upper region of medial border and superior angle of the scapula

13) Medial border of the scapula between spine of scapula and inferior angle

14) Upper portion of medial border of the scapula, across from spine of the scapula

Muscle	O	I
Levator scapula	_____	_____
Pectoralis major	_____	_____
Pectoralis minor	_____	_____
Rhomboid major	_____	_____
Rhomboid minor	_____	_____
Serratus anterior	_____	_____
Subclavius	_____	_____

Let's Palpate!

Remember - there are no right or wrong answers here

Locate and explore the **pectoralis minor** on three individuals. Then write three words that describe what you feel. (See p. 100-101 in *Trail Guide*)

Person #1 _____

_____

_____

_____

Person #2 _____

_____

_____

_____

Person #3 _____

_____

_____

_____

Biceps Brachii, Triceps Brachii and Coracobrachialis

Please answer the following questions.

1) Which head of the biceps brachii passes through the intertubercular groove? _____

2) Can you name an everyday action in which the biceps brachii's ability to supinate the forearm would come in handy?

_____

3) As you follow the biceps brachii belly proximally, it becomes deep to which muscle? _____

4) The thin sheet of fascia extending from the distal biceps brachii tendon is called the

_____.

5) The long head of the triceps brachii weaves between which two muscles before attaching at the infraglenoid tubercle?

_____   _____

6) To outline the distal tendon of the triceps brachii, which bony landmark do you want to locate?

_____

7) What action could you ask your partner to perform to feel the contraction of the long head of the triceps brachii?

_____

8) In anatomical position, the coracobrachialis is deep to which two muscles?

_____   _____

9) How can you position the shoulder to bring the belly of the coracobrachialis to a superficial position?

_____

10) To locate the belly of the coracobrachialis, from which muscle would you slide off and into the axilla?

_____

Shorten or Lengthen?

11) Passive abduction of the shoulder would _____ the coracobrachialis.

12) Passive extension of the shoulder would _____ the biceps brachii.

13) Passive flexion of the shoulder would _____ the triceps brachii.

14) Passive pronation of the forearm would _____ the biceps brachii.

Matching

Match the origin and insertion to the correct muscle.

Origins

1) Coracoid process of the scapula

2) Coracoid process of scapula, supraglenoid tubercle of scapula

3) Infraglenoid tubercle of the scapula, posterior surface of proximal half of the humerus and posterior surface of distal half of the humerus

Muscle	O	I
Biceps brachii	_____	_____
Coracobrachialis	_____	_____
Triceps brachii	_____	_____

Insertions

4) Medial surface of mid-humeral shaft

5) Olecranon process of the ulna

6) Tuberosity of the radius and aponeurosis of the biceps brachii

Let's Palpate!

Remember - there are no right or wrong answers here

Locate and explore the **triceps brachii** on three individuals. Then write three words that describe what you feel. (See p. 105-106 in *Trail Guide*)

Person #1 _____

_____

_____

_____

Person #2 _____

_____

_____

_____

Person #3 _____

_____

_____

_____

Please identify the following structures.

6) _____ :

7) _____   8) _____

1) _____

2) _____

3) _____

4) _____

5) _____

Anterior view of right shoulder

9) _____

10) _____

Color It!

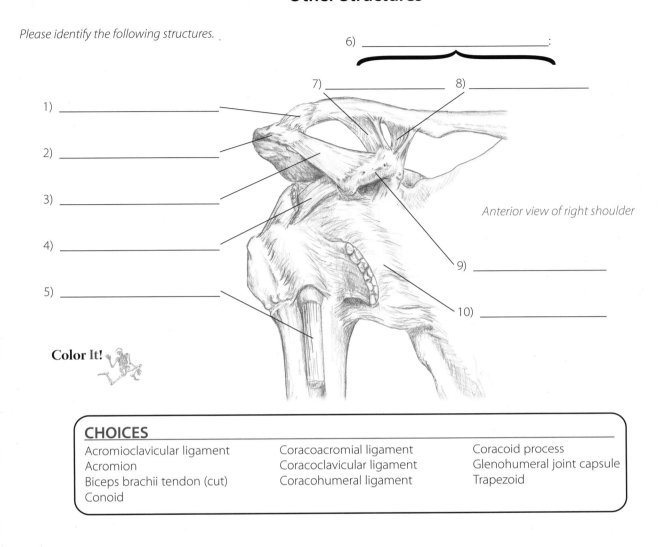

CHOICES _____

Acromioclavicular ligament   Coracoacromial ligament   Coracoid process
Acromion   Coracoclavicular ligament   Glenohumeral joint capsule
Biceps brachii tendon (cut)   Coracohumeral ligament   Trapezoid
Conoid

Please answer the following questions.

11) What should you do if your partner feels a sharp, shooting sensation down her arm while you are palpating in the axilla?

_____

12) Between which two bony landmarks can the coracoclavicular ligament be located?

_____   _____

13) The ligamentous arch that protects the rotator cuff tendons and subacromial bursa from direct trauma is formed by

the _____ ligament.

14) To bring the coracoacromial ligament closer to the surface, _____ the arm.

15) How can you position the arm to bring the subacromial bursa forward? _____

16) The brachial artery can be located on the medial side of the arm between which two muscles?

_____   _____

Please identify the following structures.

1) _____

2) _____

3) _____

4) _____

5) _____

6) _____

7) _____

8) _____

9) _____

10) _____

11) _____

12) _____

13) _____

Lateral view of right shoulder, joint opened

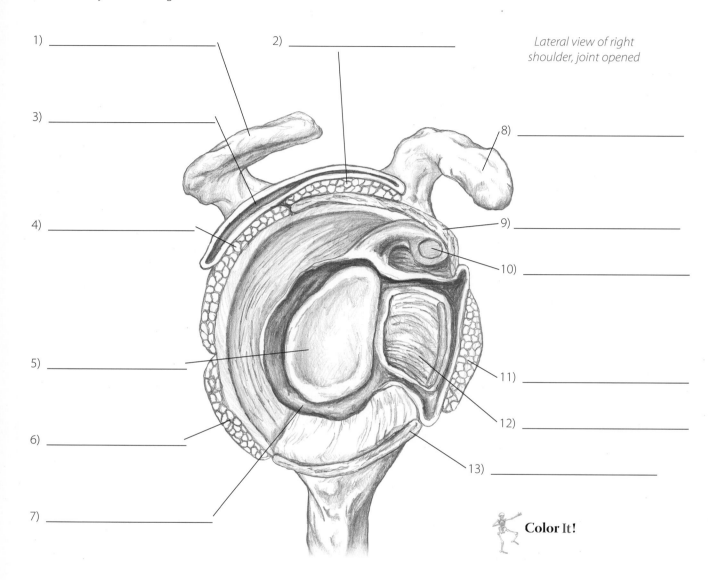

Color It!

CHOICES
Acromion
Biceps brachii tendon (long head)
Coracoid process
Glenoid cavity
Inferior glenohumeral ligament
Infraspinatus tendon
Middle glenohumeral ligament
Subacromial bursa
Subscapularis tendon
Superior glenohumeral ligament
Supraspinatus tendon
Synovial membrane
Teres minor tendon

48

Please identify the following structures.

Color It!

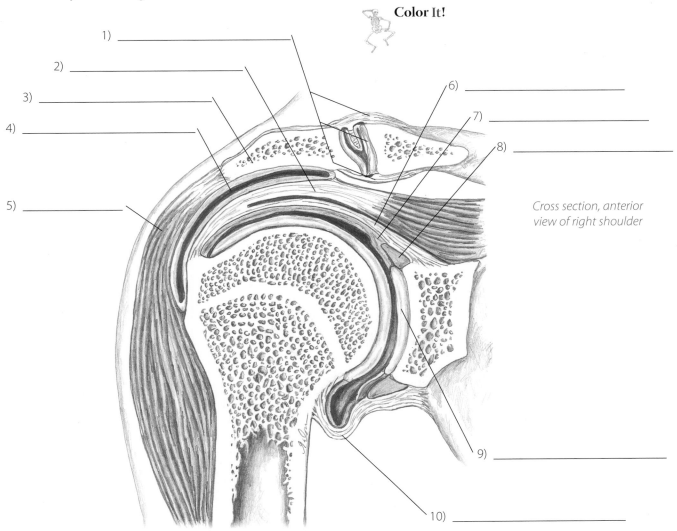

1) _____

2) _____

3) _____

4) _____

5) _____

6) _____

7) _____

8) _____

9) _____

10) _____

Cross section, anterior view of right shoulder

CHOICES

Acromioclavicular joint and ligament
Acromion
Articular capsule
Capsular ligament
Cartilage of glenoid cavity
Deltoid
Glenoid labrum
Subacromial bursa
Supraspinatus tendon
Synovial membrane

Please identify the following structures.

Color It!

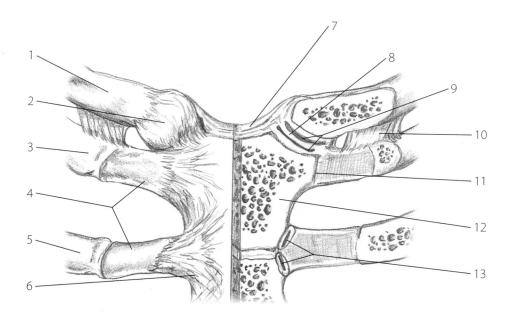

*Anterior view, right side of illustration
shown in coronal section*

1) _____

2) _____

3) _____

4) _____

5) _____

6) _____

7) _____

8) _____

9) _____

10) _____

11) _____

12) _____

13) _____

CHOICES

Anterior sternoclavicular ligament
Articular disc
Clavicle
Costal cartilages
Costoclavicular ligament
First rib
Interclavicular ligament
Joint cavity
Manubrium
Radiate sternocostal ligament
Second rib
Sternocostal joints
Sternocostal synchondrosis

50

Notes

Please identify the following structures.

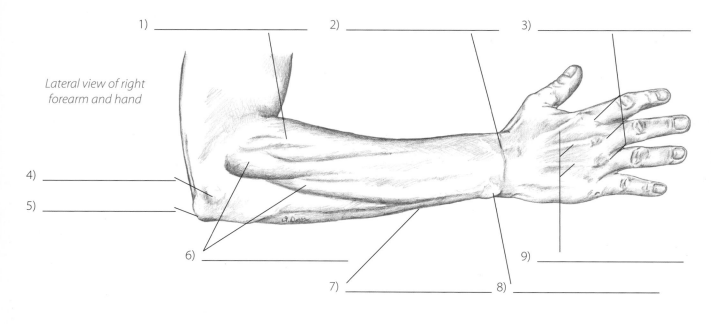

1) _____

2) _____

3) _____

Lateral view of right forearm and hand

4) _____

5) _____

6) _____

7) _____

8) _____

9) _____

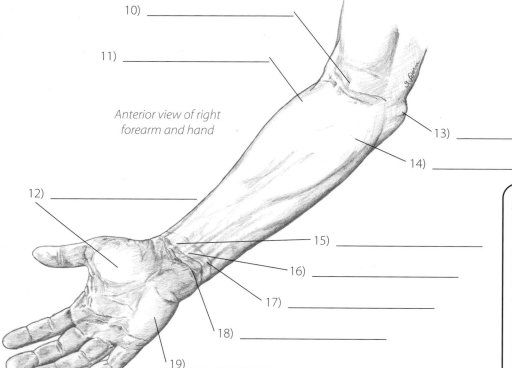

10) _____

11) _____

Anterior view of right forearm and hand

13) _____

14) _____

12) _____

15) _____

16) _____

17) _____

18) _____

19) _____

CHOICES

Biceps brachii tendon
Brachioradialis (2)
Extensor muscles
Extensor crease of the wrist
Extensor digitorum tendons
Flexor muscles
Flexor carpi radialis tendon
Flexor carpi ulnaris tendon
Flexor crease of the wrist
Head of the ulna
Hypothenar eminence
Lateral epicondyle
Medial epicondyle
Metacarpophalangeal joints
Olecranon process
Palmaris longus tendon
Shaft of the ulna
Thenar eminence

Forearm and Hand
Bones and Bony Landmarks

Please answer the following questions.

1) The palpable edge of which bone runs the length of the forearm? _____

2) Which two movements occur when the radius pivots back and forth around the ulna?

   _____   _____

3) The elbow is comprised of two joints, the _____ and _____.

4) The eight carpals are located just distal to which topographical landmark? _____

5) The olecranon process serves as an attachment site for which muscle? _____

6) Which bony landmark serves as an attachment site for the tendons of the wrist and hand extensors?

   _____

7) Which superficial, bony knob is visible along the posterior, medial side of the wrist?

   _____

8) The head of the radius is stabilized by which ligament? _____

9) Which bony landmark of the radius serves as the attachment site for brachioradialis?

   _____

10) Lister's tubercle is directly across - perhaps an inch away - from which bony landmark? _____

11) The styloid processes of the radius and ulna serve as important jumping off points for locating which group of bones?

   _____

Let's Palpate!

Remember - there are no right or wrong answers here

Locate and explore the **olecranon process and both epicondyles of the humerus** on three individuals. Then write three words that describe what you feel. (See p. 122-123 in *Trail Guide*)

Person #1 _____   Person #2 _____   Person #3 _____

_____   _____   _____

_____   _____   _____

_____   _____   _____

Please identify the following structures.

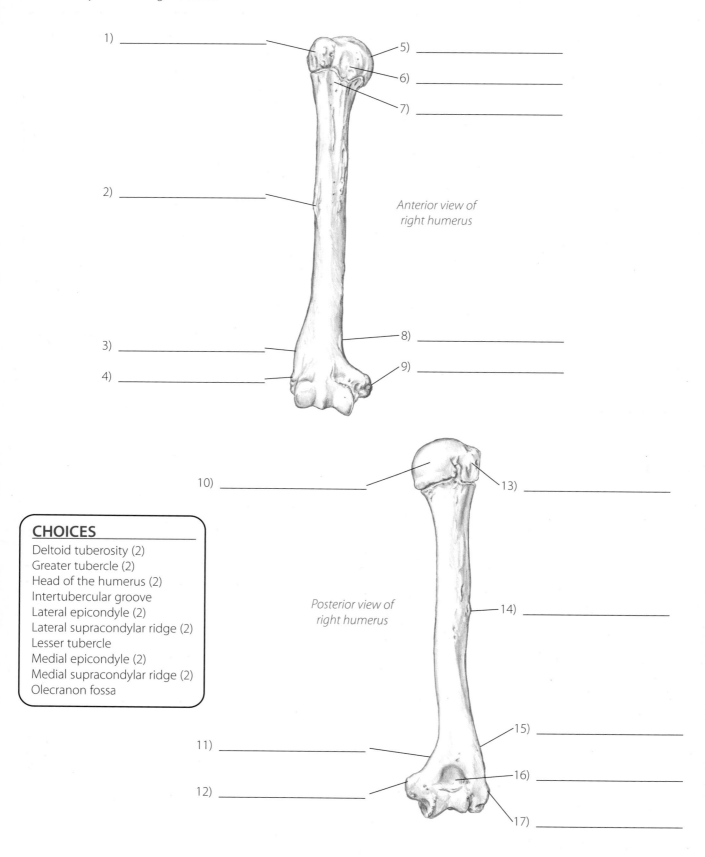

1) _____

2) _____

3) _____

4) _____

5) _____

6) _____

7) _____

8) _____

9) _____

Anterior view of right humerus

10) _____

13) _____

14) _____

Posterior view of right humerus

11) _____

12) _____

15) _____

16) _____

17) _____

CHOICES

Deltoid tuberosity (2)
Greater tubercle (2)
Head of the humerus (2)
Intertubercular groove
Lateral epicondyle (2)
Lateral supracondylar ridge (2)
Lesser tubercle
Medial epicondyle (2)
Medial supracondylar ridge (2)
Olecranon fossa

Please identify the following bones. *(Questions 1-5)*

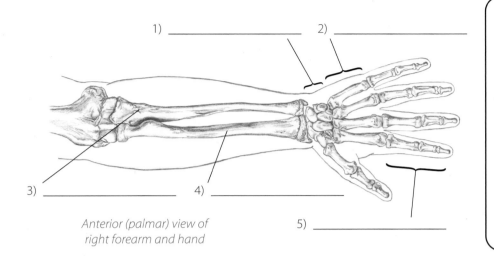

1) _____
2) _____
3) _____
4) _____
5) _____

Anterior (palmar) view of
right forearm and hand

Please identify the following bony landmarks. *(Questions 6-17)*

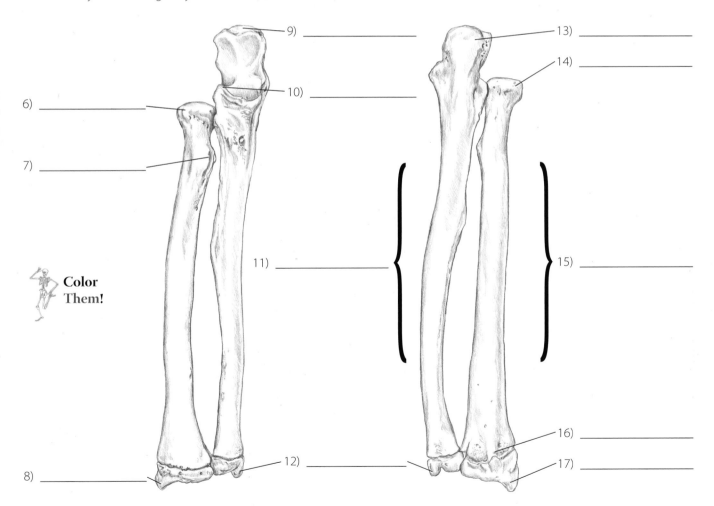

6) _____
7) _____
8) _____
9) _____
10) _____
11) _____
12) _____
13) _____
14) _____
15) _____
16) _____
17) _____

Color Them!

Anterior view of right radius and ulna   *Posterior view of right radius and ulna*

Please identify the
following structures.

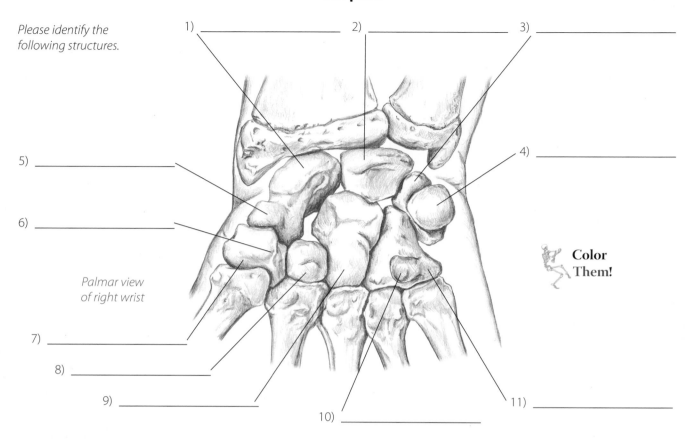

1) _____

2) _____

3) _____

4) _____

5) _____

6) _____

*Palmar view
of right wrist*

7) _____

8) _____

9) _____

10) _____

11) _____

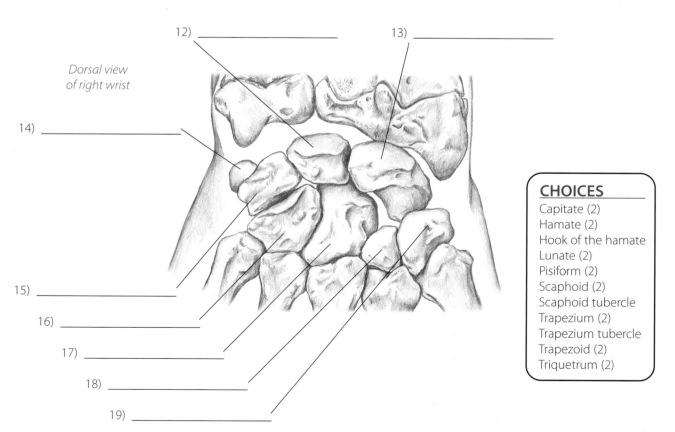

12) _____

13) _____

*Dorsal view
of right wrist*

14) _____

15) _____

16) _____

17) _____

18) _____

19) _____

CHOICES

Capitate (2)
Hamate (2)
Hook of the hamate
Lunate (2)
Pisiform (2)
Scaphoid (2)
Scaphoid tubercle
Trapezium (2)
Trapezium tubercle
Trapezoid (2)
Triquetrum (2)

Bones and Bony Landmarks of the Wrist and Hand #1

Please answer the following questions.

1) What are the four surface sides of the carpals that can be palpated?

   _____ _____ _____ _____

2) The carpals are located distal to which topographical feature of the palmar side? _____

3) Which carpal can be felt on the ulnar/palmar side of the hand, just distal to the flexor crease?

   _____

4) The pisiform acts as an attachment site for which muscle? _____

5) Which carpal can best be palpated by asking your partner to abduct and adduct her wrist as you palpate just distal

   to the styloid process of the ulna? _____

6) A hook-shaped protuberance is the distinct landmark used to isolate which carpal? _____

7) Which band of connective tissue forms the "roof" of the carpal tunnel? _____

8) Which two structures pass through the Tunnel of Guyon?

   _____ _____

9) Which four carpals serve as attachment sites for the flexor retinaculum?

   _____ _____

   _____ _____

10) Which carpal forms the floor of the "anatomical snuffbox?" _____

11) Which bone articulates with the first metacarpal and is the source of the thumb's unique movements?

   _____

12) Which carpal can be located just distal to the styloid process of the radius and felt upon adduction of the wrist?

   _____

13) Which two carpals are located between Lister's tubercle and the base of the third metacarpal and are best palpated
    from the dorsal surface?

   _____ _____

14) Anatomically speaking, the proper name for a "knuckle" joint is the _____ joint.

Extra Credit

List all eight carpal bones below. Also create your own pneumonic device to remember their order.

Please identify the following structures.

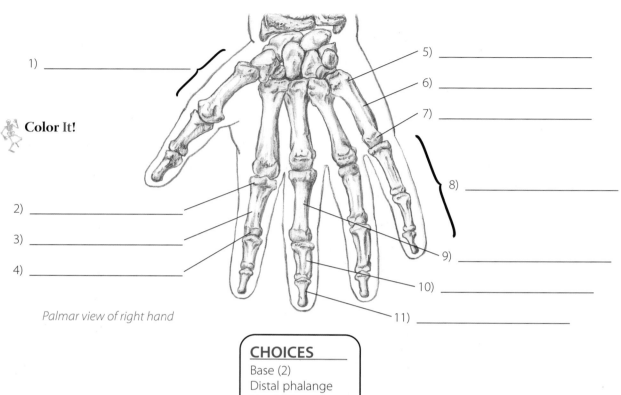

1) _____

Color It!

2) _____

3) _____

4) _____

Palmar view of right hand

5) _____

6) _____

7) _____

8) _____

9) _____

10) _____

11) _____

CHOICES

Base (2)
Distal phalange
Head (2)
Metacarpals
Middle phalange
Phalanges
Proximal phalange
Shaft (2)

Let's Palpate!

Remember - there are no right or wrong answers here

Locate and explore the **carpals** on three individuals. Then write three words that describe what you feel.
(See p. 128 in *Trail Guide*)

Person #1 _____

Person #2 _____

Person #3 _____

_____

_____

_____

_____

_____

_____

_____

_____

_____

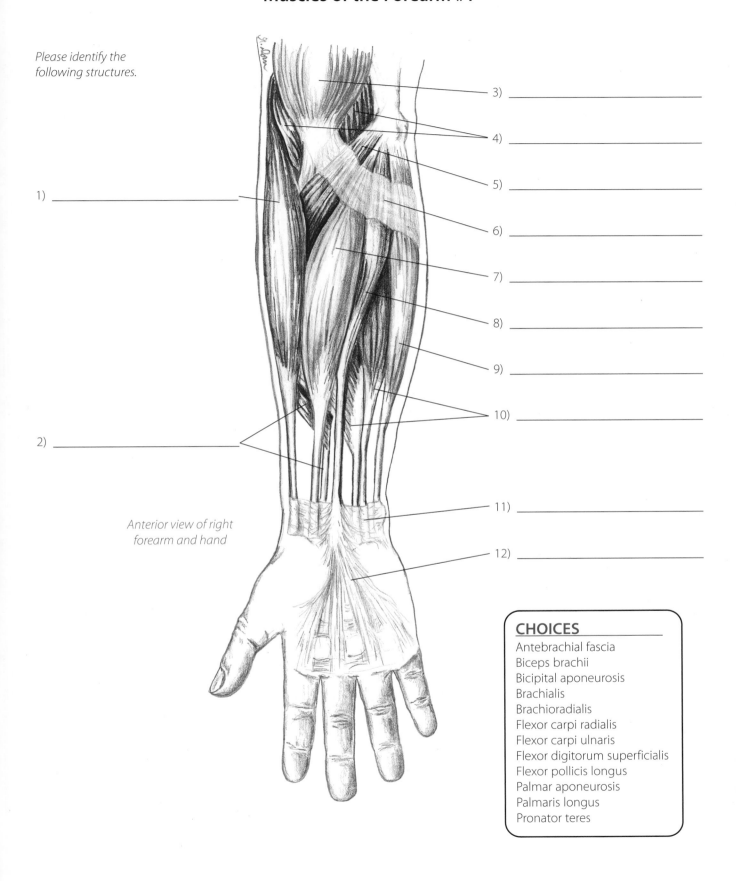

*Please identify the
following structures.*

3) _____

4) _____

5) _____

1) _____

6) _____

7) _____

8) _____

9) _____

10) _____

2) _____

11) _____

*Anterior view of right
forearm and hand*

12) _____

CHOICES

Antebrachial fascia
Biceps brachii
Bicipital aponeurosis
Brachialis
Brachioradialis
Flexor carpi radialis
Flexor carpi ulnaris
Flexor digitorum superficialis
Flexor pollicis longus
Palmar aponeurosis
Palmaris longus
Pronator teres

Please identify the following structures.

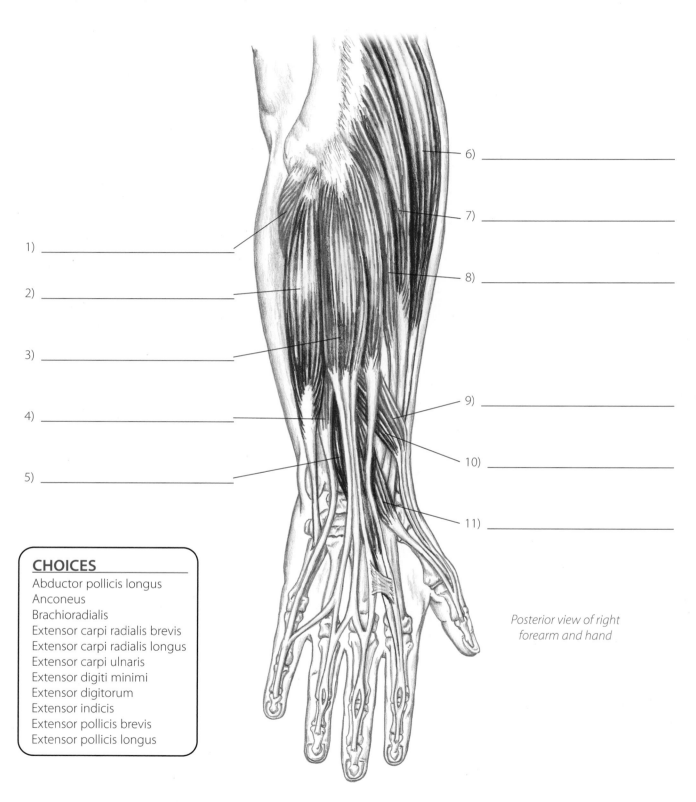

1) _____

2) _____

3) _____

4) _____

5) _____

6) _____

7) _____

8) _____

9) _____

10) _____

11) _____

*Posterior view of right
forearm and hand*

CHOICES

Abductor pollicis longus
Anconeus
Brachioradialis
Extensor carpi radialis brevis
Extensor carpi radialis longus
Extensor carpi ulnaris
Extensor digiti minimi
Extensor digitorum
Extensor indicis
Extensor pollicis brevis
Extensor pollicis longus

60

Using different colors, please fill in and label
the muscles and other structures listed below.

Antebrachial fascia
Biceps brachii
Bicipital aponeurosis
Brachialis
Brachioradialis
Flexor carpi radialis
Flexor carpi ulnaris
Flexor digitorum superficialis
Flexor pollicis longus
Palmar aponeurosis
Palmaris longus
Pronator teres

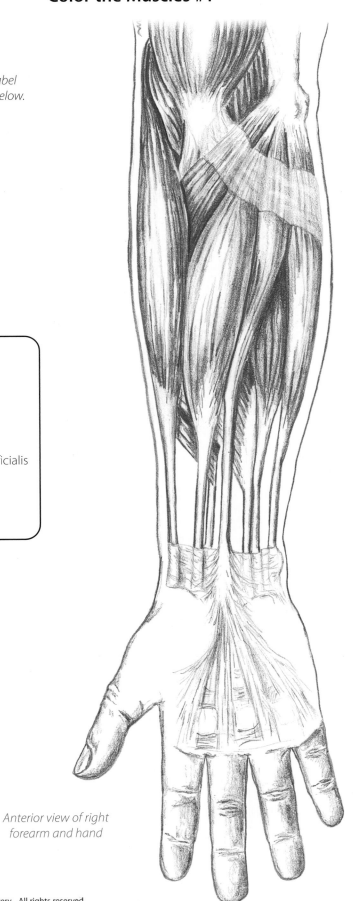

*Anterior view of right
forearm and hand*

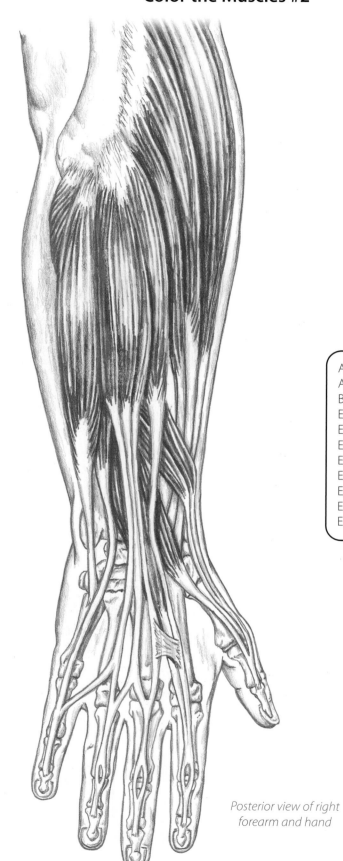

Using different colors, please fill in and label the muscles listed below.

Abductor pollicis longus
Anconeus
Brachioradialis
Extensor carpi radialis brevis
Extensor carpi radialis longus
Extensor carpi ulnaris
Extensor digiti minimi
Extensor digitorum
Extensor indicis
Extensor pollicis brevis
Extensor pollicis longus

Posterior view of right forearm and hand

Please list the action demonstrated, synergist(s) and antagonist(s).
The first letter of the muscles has been provided.

1) This action happens at which two joints?

_____

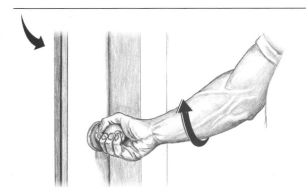

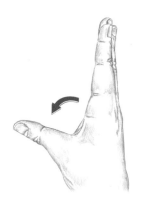

2) Action

_____

3) Synergists

B _____

S _____

4) Antagonist

P _____

7) Action

_____

8) Synergists

A _____

A _____

9) Antagonist

A _____

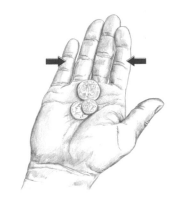

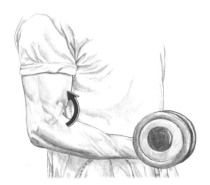

5) Action

_____

6) Muscle group that performs this action

_____

10) Action

_____

11) Synergists

F _____

P _____

12) Antagonist

T _____

1) This action happens at which joint?

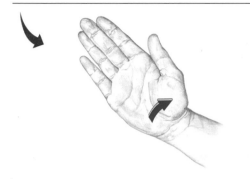

2) Action

_____

3) Synergists

E _____

F _____

4) Antagonist

E _____

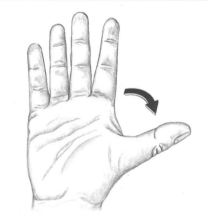

5) Action

_____

6) Synergists

E _____

A _____

7) Antagonist

F _____

Please list the action demonstrated, synergist(s) and antagonist(s). The first letter of the muscles has been provided.

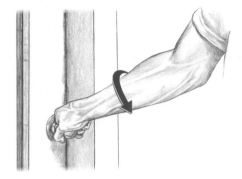

8) Action

_____

9) Synergists

P _____

B _____

10) Antagonist

B _____

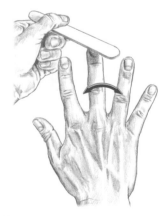

11) Action

_____

12) Muscle group that performs this action

_____

1) This action happens at which joint?

Please list the action demonstrated, two synergists and one antagonist. The first letter of the muscles has been provided.

_____

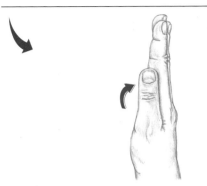

2) Action

_____

3) Synergists

A _____

P _____

4) Antagonist

A _____

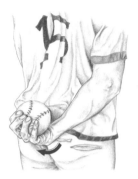

7) Action

_____

8) Synergists

F _____

F _____

9) Antagonist

E _____

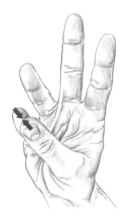

5) Action at the thumb

_____

6) Synergists

O _____

F _____

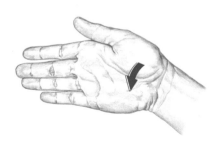

10) Action

_____

11) Synergists

E _____

F _____

12) Antagonist

F _____

Please list the action demonstrated, two synergists and one antagonist.
The first letter of the muscles has been provided.

1) This action happens at which joint?

_____

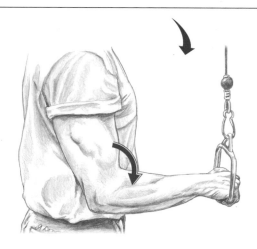

2) Action

_____

3) Synergists

T _____

A _____

4) Antagonist

B _____

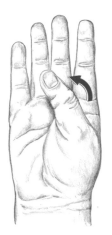

5) Action

_____

6) Synergists

F _____

A _____

7) Antagonist

A _____

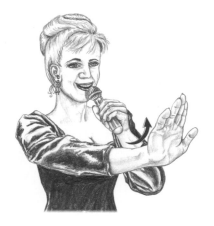

8) Action

_____

9) Synergists

E _____

E _____

10) Antagonist

P _____

Please identify the following muscles.

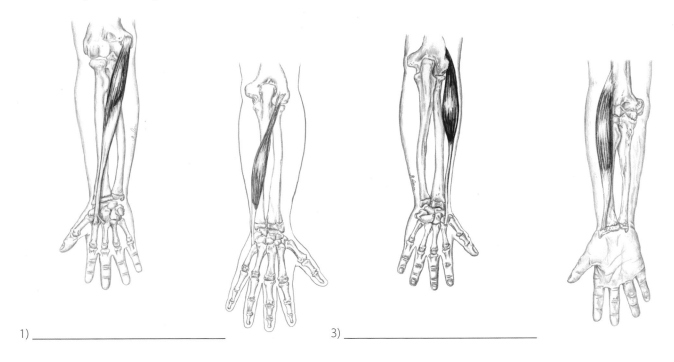

1) _____

3) _____

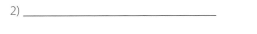

2) _____

4) _____

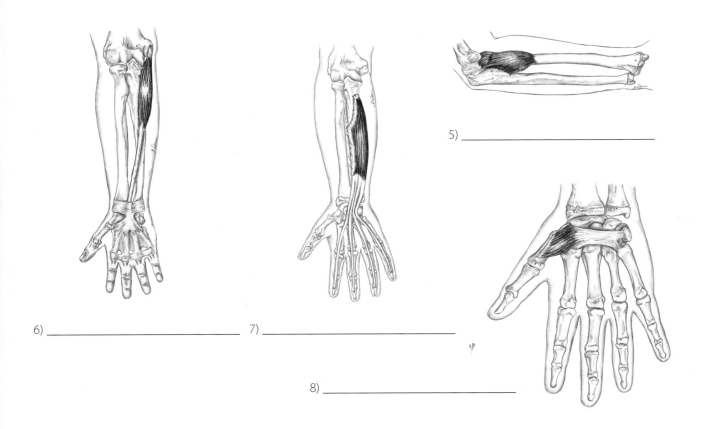

5) _____

6) _____

7) _____

8) _____

Please identify the following muscles.

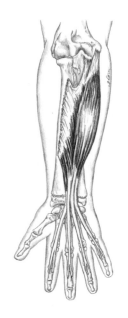

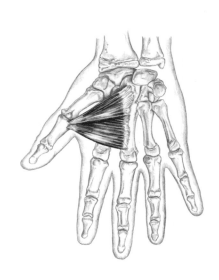

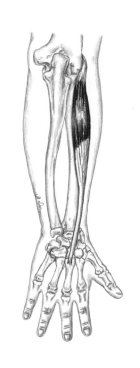

1) _____

2) _____

3) _____

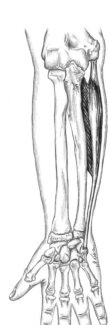

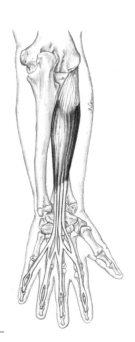

4) _____

6) _____

5) _____

7) _____

Forearm and Hand, Muscle Group #1
Brachialis, Brachioradialis, Pronators and Supinator

Please answer the following questions.

1) Which muscle is a strong elbow flexor located deep to the biceps brachii? _____

2) The brachioradialis creates a helpful dividing line between which two muscle groups?

    _____   _____

3) Which muscle runs the length of the forearm but does not cross the wrist joint? _____

4) The pronator quadratus is deep to the _____ tendons and is accessible only on the

    quadratus' _____ portion.

5) The _____ muscle is an antagonist to both the biceps brachii and supinator.

6) Palpating medial to the distal tendon of which muscle can help you locate the pronator teres?

    _____

7) To access the supinator, you must palpate deep to which muscle group? _____

Shorten or Lengthen?

8) Passive pronation of the forearm would _____ the supinator.

9) Passive flexion of the elbow would _____ the brachioradialis.

10) Passive extension of the elbow would _____ the brachialis.

11) Passive pronation of the forearm would _____ the pronator teres.

12) _____

13) _____

14) _____

15) _____

16) _____

Matching

Match the origin and insertion to the correct muscle.

Origins

1) Distal half of anterior surface of humerus

2) Lateral supracondylar ridge of humerus

3) Medial, anterior surface of distal ulna

4) Medial epicondyle of the humerus, common flexor tendon and coronoid process of the ulna

5) Radial collateral ligament, annular ligament and supinator crest of the ulna

Insertions

6) Lateral, anterior surface of distal radius

7) Lateral surface of proximal shaft of the radius

8) Middle of lateral surface of the radius

9) Styloid process of radius

10) Tuberosity and coronoid process of ulna

Muscle	O	I
Brachialis	_____	_____
Brachioradialis	_____	_____
Pronator quadratus	_____	_____
Pronator teres	_____	_____
Supinator	_____	_____

Let's Palpate!

Remember - there are no right or wrong answers here

Locate and explore the **pronator teres** on three individuals. Then write three words that describe what you feel. (See p. 154 in *Trail Guide*)

Person #1 _____

Person #2 _____

Person #3 _____

_____

_____

_____

_____

_____

_____

_____

_____

_____

Please answer the following questions.

1) With the forearm in anatomical position, the _____ group is located on the posterior/lateral side of the forearm, while the _____ group is located on the anterior/medial side.

2) The brachioradialis and the _____ clearly divide the forearm flexors from the extensors.

3) Looking at its name, what information can you gather about this muscle - *flexor carpi radialis*?

_____ _____

_____ _____

4) Which extensor muscle can be palpated alongside the shaft of the ulna? _____

5) The extensor digitorum creates movement at which fingers? _____

6) When palpating the forearm, the muscle bellies of the _____ group will feel smaller and more sinewy than the _____ group.

7) Which forearm muscles comprise the "wad of three?" _____

_____ _____

8) Which action can you ask your partner to perform at the wrist to distinguish the brachioradialis from the extensor carpi radialis? _____

9) What are the three superficial muscles in the flexor group? _____

_____ _____

10) Flexor digitorum superficialis and flexor digitorum profundus each have _____ thin tendons which pass through which anatomical structure? _____

11) Pinching the fingers together highlights the tendon of which muscle at the wrist? _____

12) What muscle runs between the pisiform and the medial epicondyle? _____

13) Although the flexor digitorum superficialis and profundus are deep to the other forearm flexors, they can be accessed along the medial side of which bony landmark? _____

Let's Palpate! *Remember - there are no right or wrong answers here*

Locate and explore the **extensor digitorum** on three individuals. Then write three words that describe what you feel. (See p. 146 in *Trail Guide*)

Person #1 _____ Person #2 _____ Person #3 _____

_____ _____ _____

_____ _____ _____

_____ _____ _____

Matching

Match the origin and insertion to the correct muscle.

Origins

1) Anterior and medial surfaces of proximal three-quarters of ulna

2) Common extensor tendon from the lateral epicondyle of humerus (2)

3) Common flexor tendon from medial epicondyle (3)

4) Common flexor tendon from medial epicondyle, ulnar collateral ligament, coronoid process of ulna and shaft of radius

5) Lateral supracondylar ridge of humerus (2)

Insertions

6) Base of fifth metacarpal

7) Bases of second and third metacarpals

8) Base of second metacarpal

9) Base of third metacarpal

10) By four tendons into bases of distal phalanges, palmar surface of second through fifth fingers

11) By four tendons into sides of middle phalanges of second through fifth fingers

12) Flexor retinaculum and palmar aponeurosis

13) Middle and distal phalanges of second through fifth fingers

14) Pisiform

Muscle	O	I
Extensor carpi radialis brevis	_____	_____
Extensor carpi radialis longus	_____	_____
Extensor carpi ulnaris	_____	_____
Extensor digitorum	_____	_____
Flexor carpi radialis	_____	_____
Flexor carpi ulnaris	_____	_____
Flexor digitorum profundus	_____	_____
Flexor digitorum superficialis	_____	_____
Palmaris longus	_____	_____

Shorten or Lengthen?

15) Passive abduction of the wrist would _____ the extensor carpi radialis longus.

16) Passive flexion of fingers 2-5 would _____ the extensor digitorum.

17) Passive flexion of the wrist would _____ the palmaris longus.

18) Passive adduction of the wrist would _____ the flexor carpi radialis.

19) Passive extension of fingers 2-5 would _____ the flexor digitorum profundus.

Please answer the following questions.

1) The _____ eminence is located at the thumb's base, while the

   _____ eminence is located along the ulnar side of the palm.

2) How many muscles act upon the thumb? _____

   How many of these are located at the thenar eminence? _____

3) Which muscle is responsible for creating opposition of the thumb? _____

4) The distal tendons of which three muscles form the "anatomical snuffbox?"

   _____   _____   _____

5) The palmar interossei are difficult to access because they are deep to the _____

   muscles and situated between the _____ bones.

6) The lumbricals sprout from the sides of the tendons of which muscle? _____

7) Which muscle is located between the pisiform and the base of the fifth finger? _____

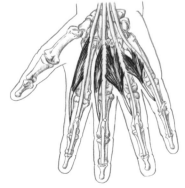

8) _____

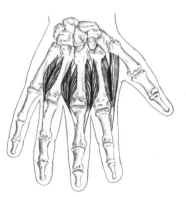

9) _____

10) _____

11) _____

Matching

Match the origin and insertion to the correct muscle.

Origins

1) Anterior surface of radius and interosseous membrane

2) Capitate, second and third metacarpals

3) Flexor retinaculum and tubercle of the trapezium

4) Posterior surface of radius and ulna, and interosseous membrane

5) Posterior surface of ulna and interosseous membrane

Insertions

6) Base of first metacarpal

7) Base of proximal phalange of thumb

8) Distal phalange of thumb (2)

9) Entire length of first metacarpal bone, radial side

Muscle	O	I
Abductor pollicis longus	_____	_____
Adductor pollicis	_____	_____
Extensor pollicis longus	_____	_____
Flexor pollicis longus	_____	_____
Opponens pollicis	_____	_____

Let's Palpate!

Remember - there are no right or wrong answers here

Locate and explore the **thenar eminence** on three individuals. Then write three words that describe what you feel. (See p. 159 in *Trail Guide*)

Person #1 _____

Person #2 _____

Person #3 _____

_____

_____

_____

_____

_____

_____

_____

_____

_____

Forearm and Hand
Other Structures

Please answer the following questions.

1) Which two structures reinforce the elbow joint by spanning from their respective epicondyles to the bones of the forearm?

   _____   _____

2) During pronation and supination, which ligament stabilizes the proximal end of the radius against the ulna?

   _____

3) Between which two bony landmarks is the ulnar nerve particularly accessible and superficial?

   _____   _____

4) Which structure pads the space between the olecranon process and the skin of the elbow?

   _____

5) The carpal tunnel is a passageway for many _____ and the _____ nerve.

6) The transverse fibers of the _____ and carpal bones form the carpal tunnel.

7) Which span of connective tissue is a continuation of the antebrachial fascia into the palm of the hand?

   _____

8) Which artery is often used for taking a pulse at the wrist? _____

---

10) _____

Please identify the following structures.

9) _____

11) _____

Cross section of right wrist

Color It!

13) _____

12) _____

Please identify the following structures.

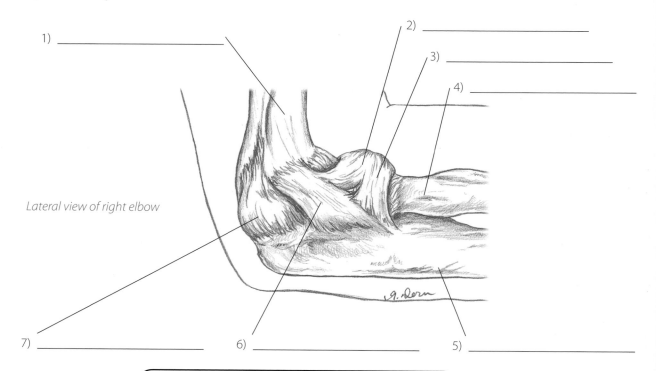

1) _____

2) _____

3) _____

4) _____

Lateral view of right elbow

7) _____

6) _____

5) _____

CHOICES

Annular ligament (2)	Olecranon process
Articular capsule (2)	Radial collateral ligament
Head of radius (deep)	Radius (2)
Humerus (2)	Ulna (2)
Medial epicondyle	Ulnar collateral ligament

Color Them!

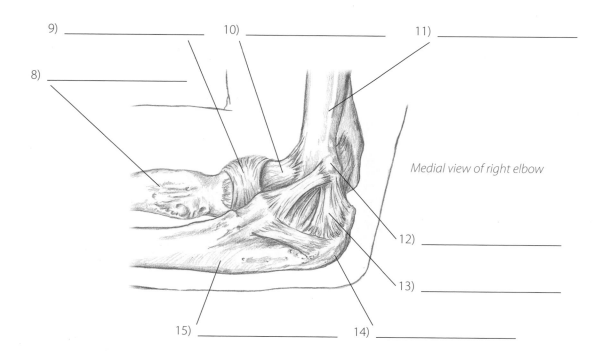

9) _____

10) _____

11) _____

8) _____

Medial view of right elbow

12) _____

13) _____

15) _____

14) _____

Please identify the following structures.

1) _____ :

2) _____

3) _____

4) _____

5) _____

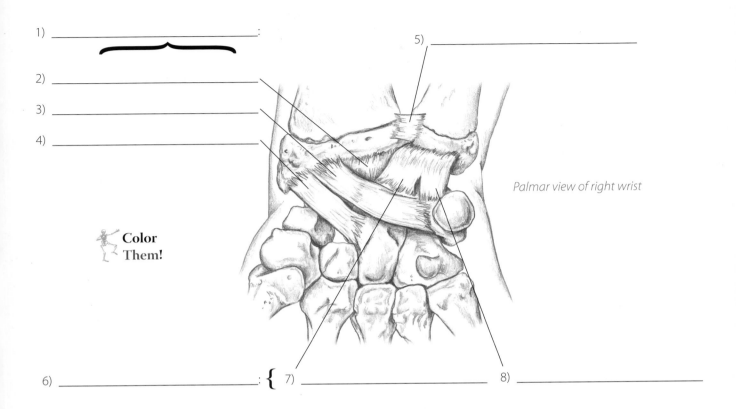

Palmar view of right wrist

Color Them!

6) _____ : { 7) _____   8) _____

CHOICES

Dorsal radiocarpal ligament
Dorsal radioulnar ligament
Palmar radiocarpal ligament
Palmar radioulnar ligament
Palmar ulnocarpal ligament
Radial collateral ligament
Radiocapite part
Radioscapholunate part
Radiotriquetral part
Ulnar collateral ligament
Ulnolunate part
Ulnotriquetral part

9) _____   10) _____

11) _____

12) _____

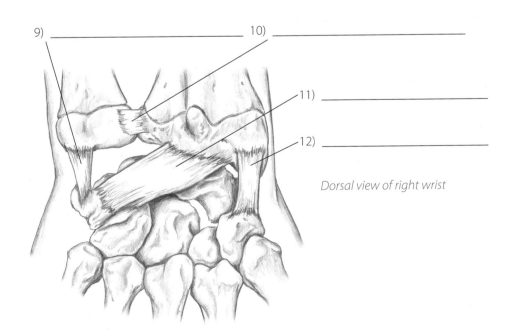

Dorsal view of right wrist

Please identify the following structures.

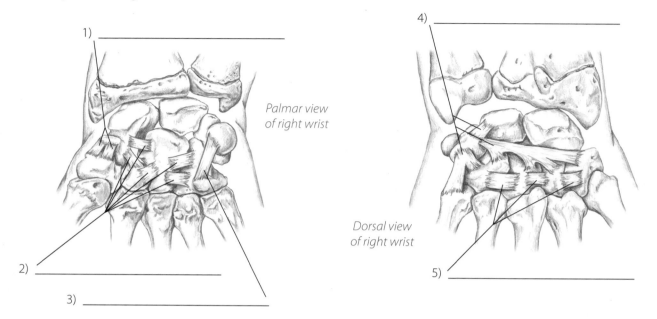

1) _____

*Palmar view
of right wrist*

2) _____

3) _____

4) _____

*Dorsal view
of right wrist*

5) _____

**Color
Them!**

CHOICES

Distal intercarpal ligaments
Dorsal carpometacarpal ligaments
Dorsal intercarpal ligaments
Dorsal metacarpal ligaments
Palmar carpometacarpal ligaments

Palmar intercarpal ligaments
Palmar metacarpal ligaments
Pisohamate ligament
Pisometacarpal ligament
Radiate carpal ligaments

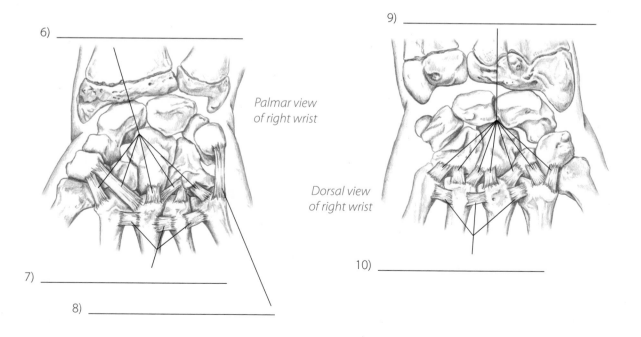

6) _____

*Palmar view
of right wrist*

7) _____

8) _____

9) _____

*Dorsal view
of right wrist*

10) _____

Notes

Please identify the following structures.

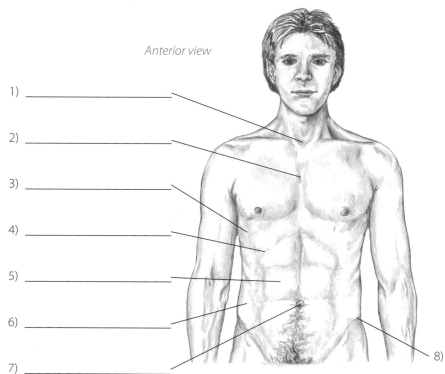

Anterior view

1) _____

2) _____

3) _____

4) _____

5) _____

6) _____

7) _____

8) _____

CHOICES

Edge of rib cage
Erector spinae group
External oblique
Iliac crest (2)
Jugular notch
Medial border of the scapula
Posterior superior iliac spine
Rectus abdominis
Ribs
Sacrum
Spinous process of C-7
Spinous processes of thoracic
    and lumbar vertebrae
Sternum
Twelfth rib
Umbilicus

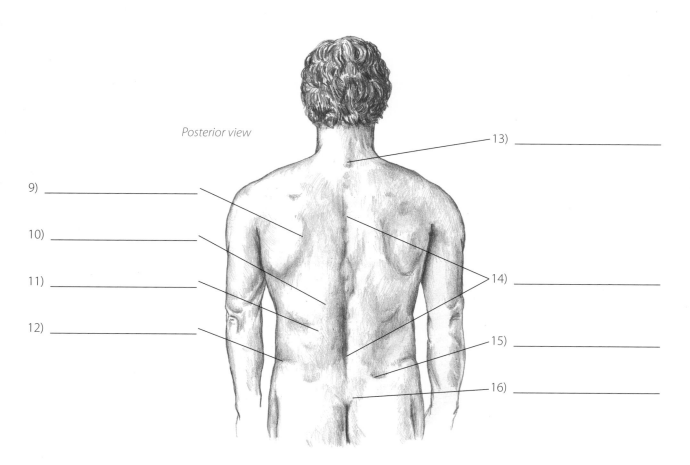

Posterior view

9) _____

10) _____

11) _____

12) _____

13) _____

14) _____

15) _____

16) _____

80

Please answer the following questions.

1) Which section of the vertebral column is capable of the most movement? _____

2) The thorax is comprised of which two structures?

_____   _____

3) The visible row of bumps running down the center of the back are the _____.

4) Please match the bony landmark with the corresponding spinous process.

_____ T-12   a) Top of the iliac crest

_____ T-2   b) Base of the neck

_____ L-4   c) Superior angle of the scapula

_____ C-7   d) Twelfth rib

_____ T-7   e) Inferior angle of the scapula

5) With your partner seated, what two movements at the spine could you ask your partner to perform to feel the movement of the spinous processes?

_____   _____

6) The angles of the scapula and the corresponding spinous processes do not always line up. Name two factors that might affect the position of the scapula.

_____   _____

7) Which two cervical vertebrae have spinous processes that protrude further posteriorly and are more distinct than the other cervical vertebrae?

_____   _____

8) Which band of connective tissue lies superficial to the cervical spinous processes?

_____

9) Many of the cervical transverse processes are deep to which neck muscle? _____

10) Your partner is supine and you passively rotate the head 45° away from the side you are palpating. This position places the cervical transverse processes in a line running between which two bony landmarks?

_____   _____

11) The lamina groove is located between which two bony landmarks of the vertebrae?

_____   _____

Please answer the following questions.

1) The thoracic transverse processes are located deep to the _____ muscles and superficial to the _____.

2) To avoid the thick erector spinae muscles overlying the lumbar transverse processes, it is best to slide your fingers roughly how far laterally from the spinous processes? _____

3) Which rib attaches to the sternum at the level of the sternal angle? _____

4) What is the structure that extends off the ribs and attaches to the sternum? _____

5) Which muscles are located between the ribs? _____

6) Although the entire rib cage is deep to muscle tissue, which portion is easily accessed?

    _____

7) The first rib is deep to which bone along the anterior thorax? _____

8) Exploring just posterior to the clavicle, through which muscle group must you palpate to access the first rib?

    _____

9) What action could you ask your partner to perform to feel the first rib move? _____

10) In which three directions are the ribs ideally designed to move? _____

    _____   _____

11) The eleventh and twelfth ribs lie at approximately what angle on the body? _____

12) As you palpate medially toward the spine, you may lose contact with the twelfth rib because it is deep to which muscle group?

    _____

Let's Palpate!

Remember - there are no right or wrong answers here

Locate and explore the **spinous processes of the vertebral column** on three individuals. Then write three words that describe what you feel. (See p. 182 in *Trail Guide*)

Person #1 _____   Person #2 _____   Person #3 _____

_____   _____   _____

_____   _____   _____

_____   _____   _____

Please identify the following structures.

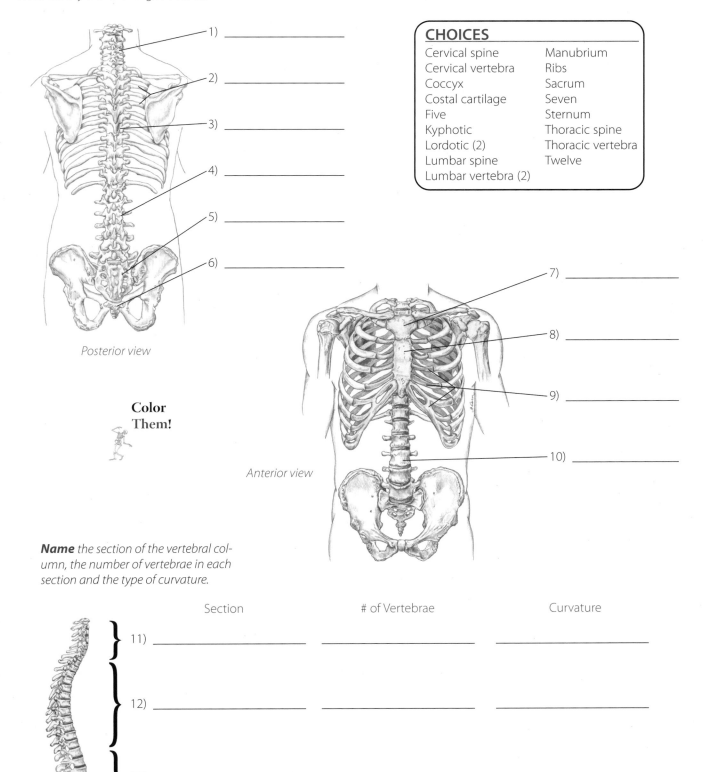

1) _____

2) _____

3) _____

4) _____

5) _____

6) _____

CHOICES

Cervical spine	Manubrium
Cervical vertebra	Ribs
Coccyx	Sacrum
Costal cartilage	Seven
Five	Sternum
Kyphotic	Thoracic spine
Lordotic (2)	Thoracic vertebra
Lumbar spine	Twelve
Lumbar vertebra (2)	

Posterior view

Color Them!

7) _____

8) _____

9) _____

10) _____

Anterior view

Name *the section of the vertebral column, the number of vertebrae in each
section and the type of curvature.*

	Section	# of Vertebrae	Curvature
11)	_____	_____	_____
12)	_____	_____	_____
13)	_____	_____	_____

Lateral view

Please identify the following structures.

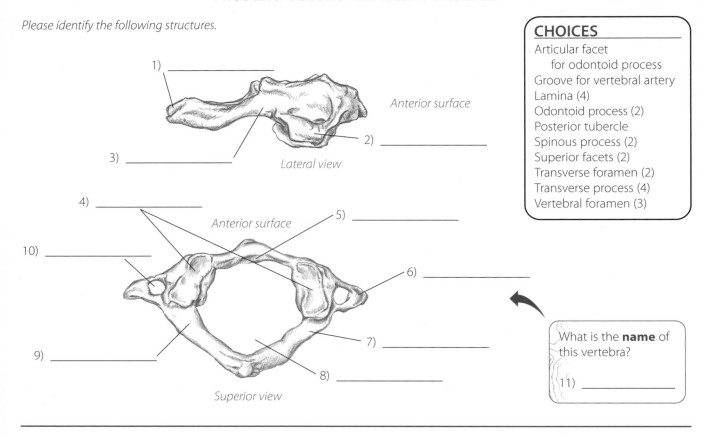

1) _____

Anterior surface

2) _____

3) _____

Lateral view

4) _____

Anterior surface

5) _____

10) _____

6) _____

9) _____

7) _____

8) _____

Superior view

What is the **name** of this vertebra?

11) _____

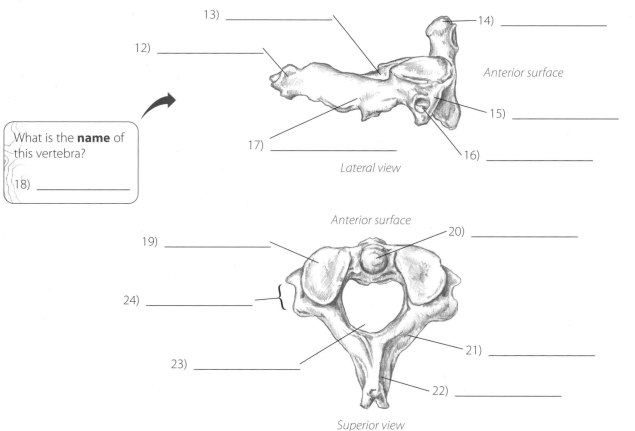

13) _____

14) _____

12) _____

Anterior surface

15) _____

17) _____

16) _____

Lateral view

What is the **name** of this vertebra?

18) _____

Anterior surface

19) _____

20) _____

24) _____

21) _____

23) _____

22) _____

Superior view

84

Please identify the following structures.

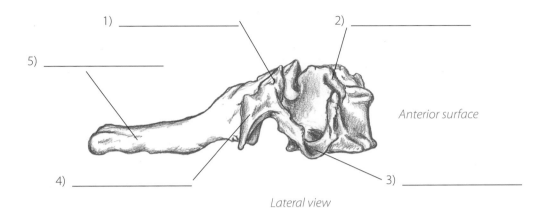

1) _____

2) _____

5) _____

Anterior surface

4) _____

3) _____

Lateral view

CHOICES

Anterior tubercle (2)	Posterior tubercle (2)
Body	Spinous process (2)
Canal for spinal nerve (2)	Superior facet
Lamina	Transverse foramen
Lamina groove	Transverse process (2)

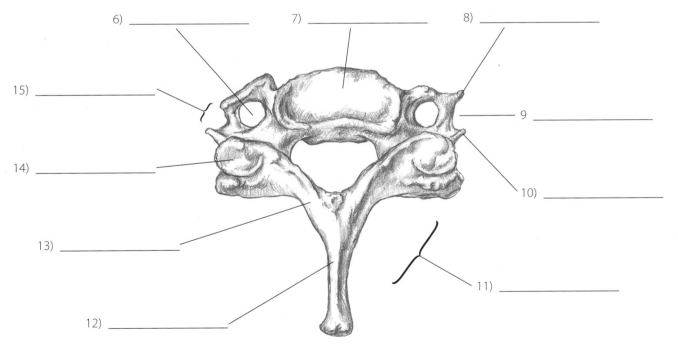

6) _____

7) _____

8) _____

15) _____

9 _____

14) _____

10) _____

13) _____

11) _____

12) _____

Superior view

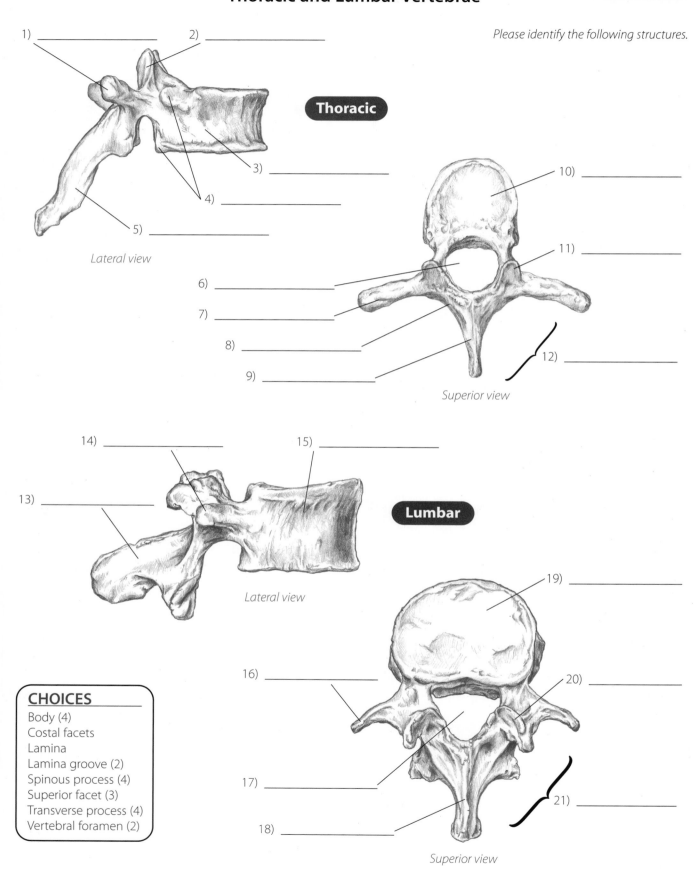

1) _____   2) _____

Please identify the following structures.

Thoracic

3) _____

4) _____

5) _____

Lateral view

10) _____

11) _____

6) _____

7) _____

8) _____

9) _____

12) _____

Superior view

14) _____   15) _____

13) _____

Lumbar

Lateral view

19) _____

16) _____

20) _____

17) _____

18) _____

21) _____

Superior view

CHOICES
Body (4)
Costal facets
Lamina
Lamina groove (2)
Spinous process (4)
Superior facet (3)
Transverse process (4)
Vertebral foramen (2)

Please identify the following structures.

1) _____

2) _____

3) _____

4) _____

5) _____

6) _____

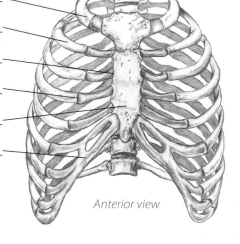

Anterior view

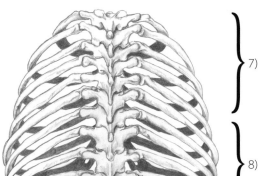

7) _____

8) _____

9) _____

Posterior view

Color Them!

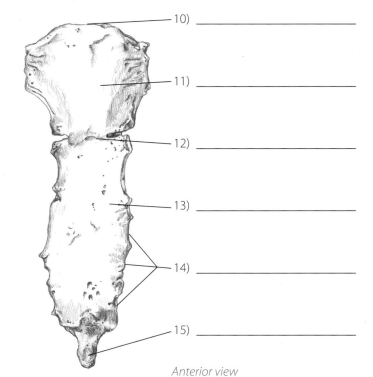

10) _____

11) _____

12) _____

13) _____

14) _____

15) _____

Anterior view

CHOICES

Articulations with ribs	Manubrium
Body of sternum	Second rib
Costal cartilage	Sternal angle
Costochondral joint	Sternocostal joint
False ribs	Sternum
First rib	True ribs
Floating ribs	Xiphoid process
Jugular notch	

Please identify the following structures.

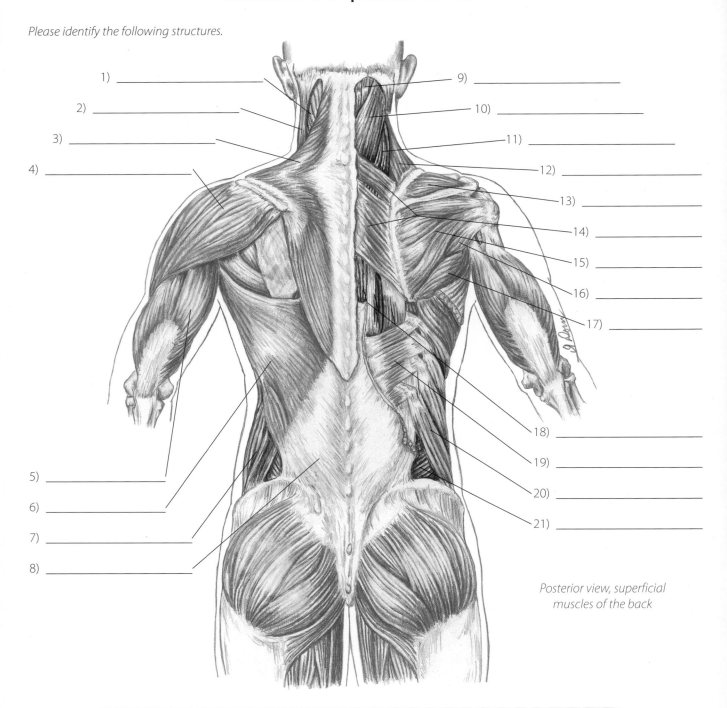

1) _____

2) _____

3) _____

4) _____

5) _____

6) _____

7) _____

8) _____

9) _____

10) _____

11) _____

12) _____

13) _____

14) _____

15) _____

16) _____

17) _____

18) _____

19) _____

20) _____

21) _____

Posterior view, superficial muscles of the back

CHOICES

Deltoid	Rhomboids	Supraspinatus
Erector spinae group	Semispinalis capitis	Teres major
External oblique (2)	Serratus posterior inferior	Teres minor
Infraspinatus	Splenius capitis (2)	Thoracolumbar aponeurosis
Internal oblique	Splenius cervicis	Trapezius
Latissimus dorsi	Sternocleidomastoid	Triceps brachii
Levator scapula		

Please identify the following structures.

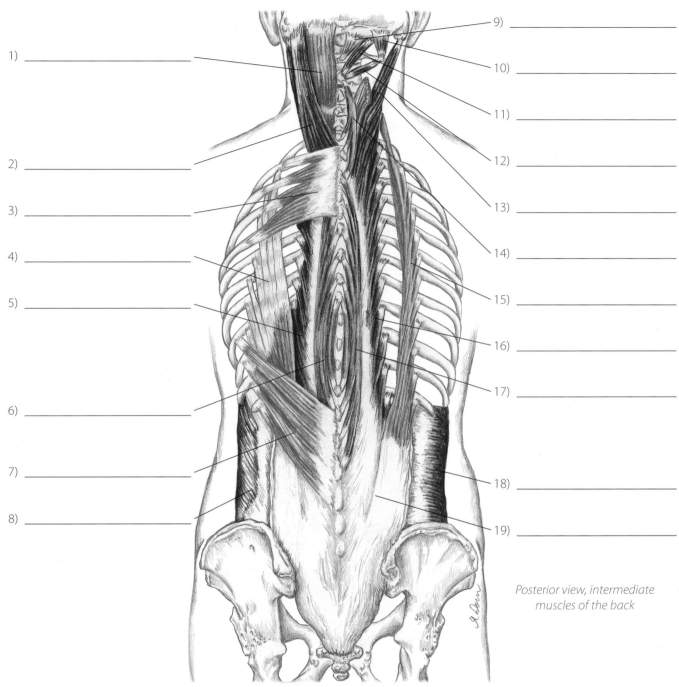

Posterior view, intermediate muscles of the back

1) _____

2) _____

3) _____

4) _____

5) _____

6) _____

7) _____

8) _____

9) _____

10) _____

11) _____

12) _____

13) _____

14) _____

15) _____

16) _____

17) _____

18) _____

19) _____

CHOICES

Iliocostalis (2)	Rectus capitis posterior major	Spinalis cervicis
Internal oblique	Rectus capitis posterior minor	Spinalis thoracis (2)
Longissimus capitis	Semispinalis capitis	Splenius capitis
Longissimus thoracis (2)	Serratus posterior inferior	Thoracolumbar aponeurosis
Oblique capitis inferior	Serratus posterior superior	Transverse abdominis
Oblique capitis superior		

Please identify the
following structures.

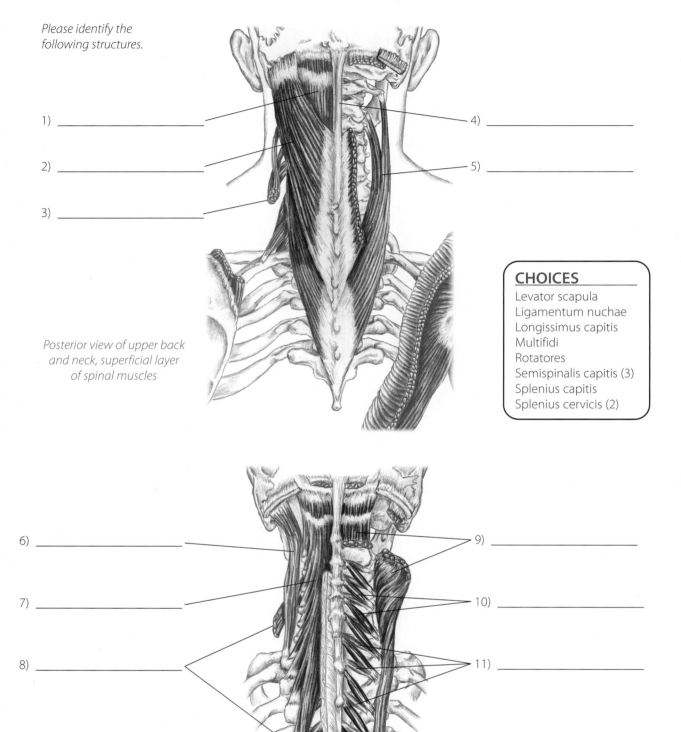

1) _____

2) _____

3) _____

4) _____

5) _____

*Posterior view of upper back
and neck, superficial layer
of spinal muscles*

CHOICES

Levator scapula
Ligamentum nuchae
Longissimus capitis
Multifidi
Rotatores
Semispinalis capitis (3)
Splenius capitis
Splenius cervicis (2)

6) _____

7) _____

8) _____

9) _____

10) _____

11) _____

*Posterior view of upper back and neck,
intermediate layer of spinal muscles*

Please identify the following structures.

Color It!

Anterior surface

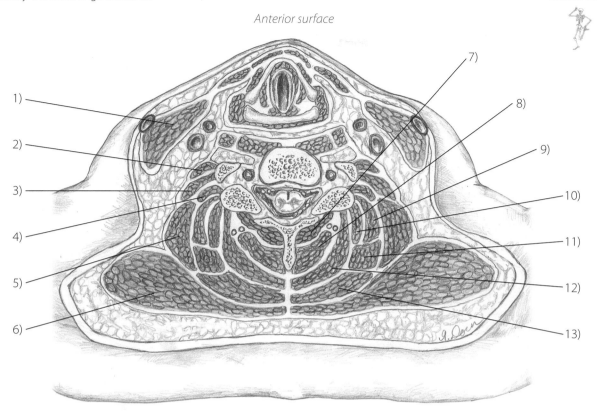

Cross section of the neck at the level of the fifth cervical vertebra

---

CHOICES

Anterior scalene	Semispinalis capitis
Levator scapula	Semispinalis cervicis
Longissimus capitis	Splenius capitis
Longissimus cervicis	Splenius cervicis
Middle scalene	Sternocleidomastoid
Multifidi and spinalis cervicis	Trapezius
Posterior scalene	

1) _____

2) _____

3) _____

4) _____

5) _____

6) _____

7) _____

8) _____

9) _____

10) _____

11) _____

12) _____

13) _____

Please identify the following structures.

Color It!

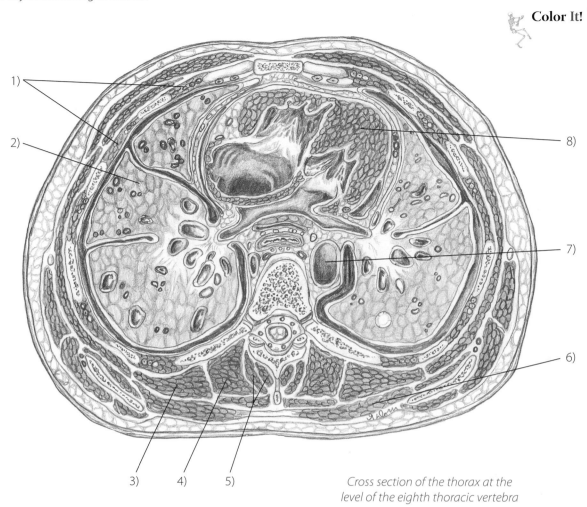

1)
2)
8)
7)
6)
3)   4)   5)

Cross section of the thorax at the level of the eighth thoracic vertebra

CHOICES
Abdominal aorta
Heart
Iliocostalis
Intercostals
Longissimus
Lung
Multifidi and rotatores
Trapezius

1) _____

2) _____

3) _____

4) _____

5) _____

6) _____

7) _____

8) _____

Please identify the following structures.

Color It!

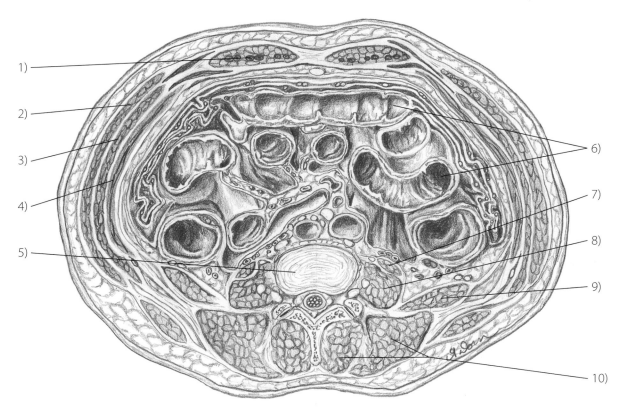

Cross section of the thorax at the level of the third lumbar vertebra

CHOICES

Body of L-3
Erector spinae group
External oblique
Internal oblique
Intestines

Psoas major
Psoas minor
Quadratus lumborum
Rectus abdominis
Transverse abdominis

1) _____

2) _____

3) _____

4) _____

5) _____

6) _____

7) _____

8) _____

9) _____

10) _____

Using different colors, please fill in and label the muscles and other structures listed below.

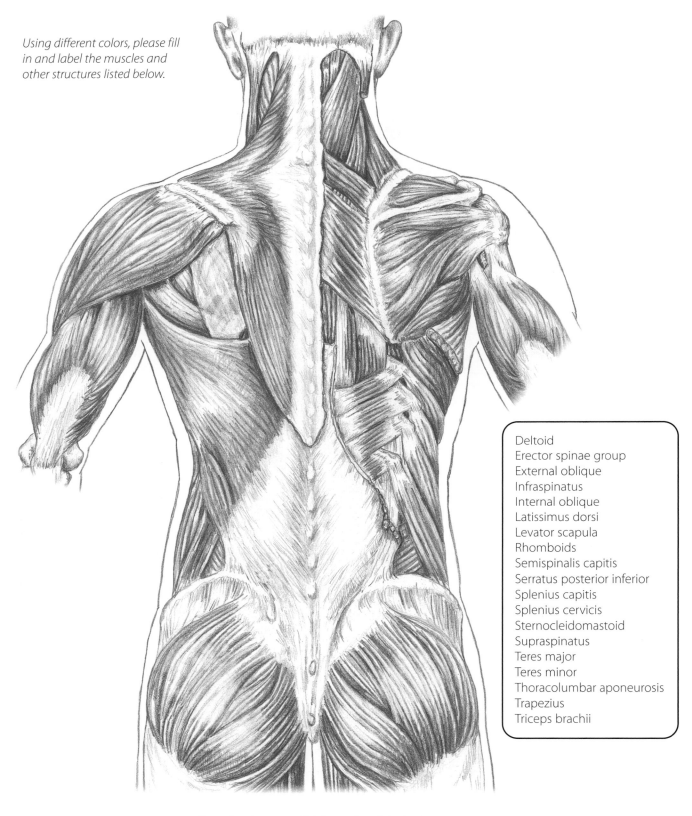

Deltoid
Erector spinae group
External oblique
Infraspinatus
Internal oblique
Latissimus dorsi
Levator scapula
Rhomboids
Semispinalis capitis
Serratus posterior inferior
Splenius capitis
Splenius cervicis
Sternocleidomastoid
Supraspinatus
Teres major
Teres minor
Thoracolumbar aponeurosis
Trapezius
Triceps brachii

Posterior view, superficial muscles of the back

Using different colors, please fill in and label the muscles and other structures listed below.

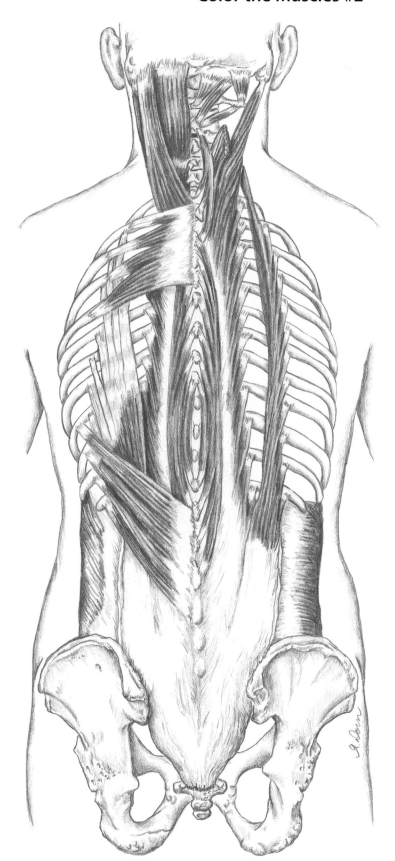

Posterior view, intermediate muscles of the back

Iliocostalis
Internal oblique
Longissimus
Longissimus capitis
Oblique capitis inferior
Oblique capitis superior
Rectus capitis posterior major
Rectus capitis posterior minor
Semispinalis capitis
Serratus posterior inferior
Serratus posterior superior
Spinalis
Spinalis cervicis
Splenius capitis
Thoracolumbar aponeurosis
Transverse abdominis

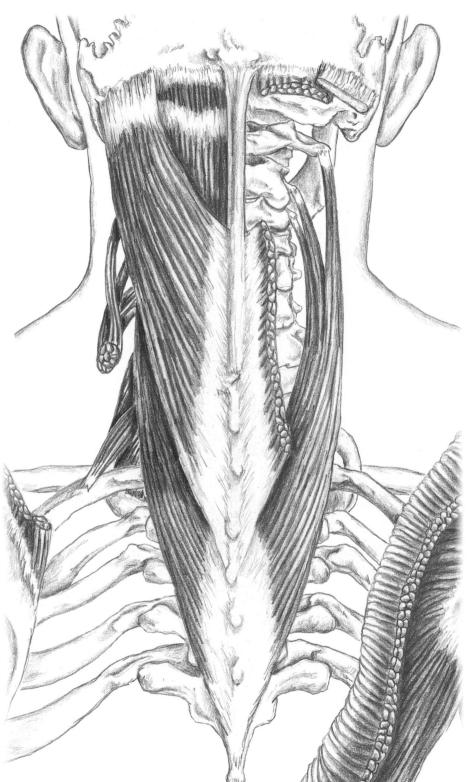

Using different colors, please fill in and label the muscles and other structures listed below.

Levator scapula (cut)
Ligamentum nuchae
Semispinalis capitis
Splenius capitis
Splenius cervicis
Trapezius
   (cut and reflected)

Posterior view of upper back and neck, superficial layer of spinal muscles

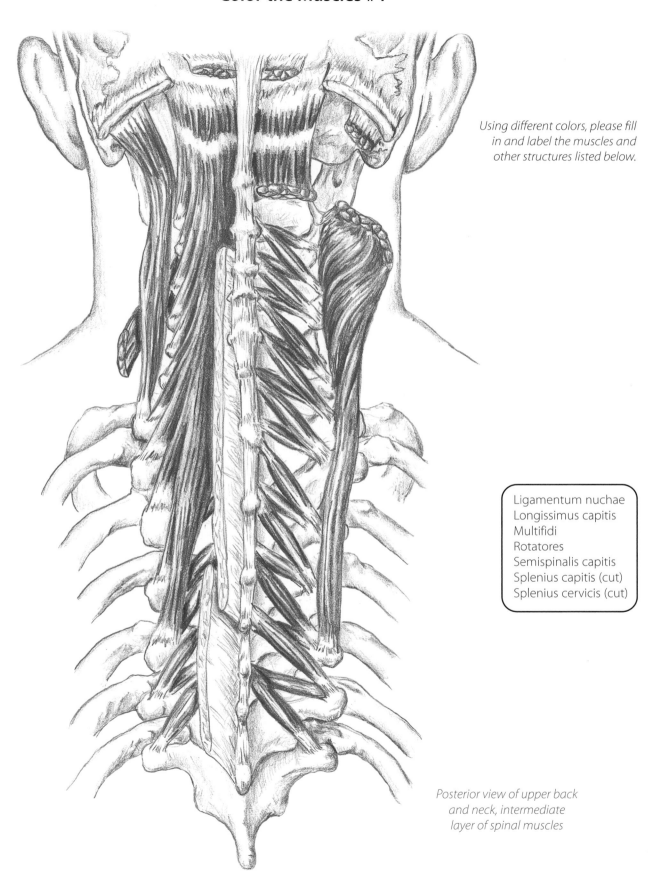

Using different colors, please fill in and label the muscles and other structures listed below.

Ligamentum nuchae
Longissimus capitis
Multifidi
Rotatores
Semispinalis capitis
Splenius capitis (cut)
Splenius cervicis (cut)

Posterior view of upper back and neck, intermediate layer of spinal muscles

Please list the action demonstrated, two synergists and one antagonist.
The first letter of the muscles has been provided.

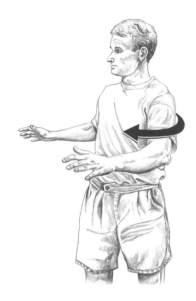

1) Action (to his right)

_____

2) Synergists (and on what side - his left or right?)

E _____

I _____

3) Antagonist (and on what side - his left or right?)

M _____

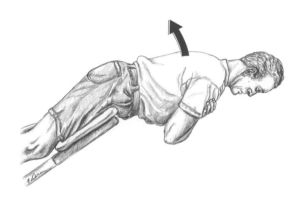

4) Action

_____

5) Synergists

S _____

I _____

6) Antagonist

R _____

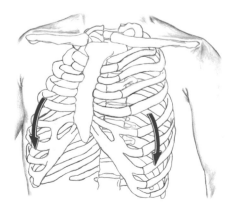

7) Action

_____

8) Synergists

I _____

S _____

9) Antagonist

E _____

Please list the action demonstrated, two synergists and one antagonist.
The first letter of the muscles has been provided.

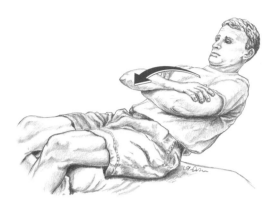

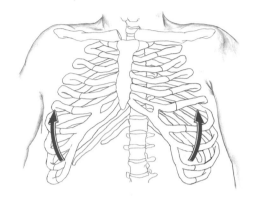

1) Action

_____

2) Synergists

E _____

I _____

3) Antagonist

Q _____

4) Action

_____

5) Synergists

S _____

S _____

6) Antagonist

I _____

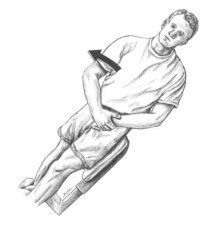

7) Action

_____

8) Synergists (and on what side - his left or right?)

Q _____

E _____

9) Antagonist (and on what side - his left or right?)

S _____

Please identify the following muscles.

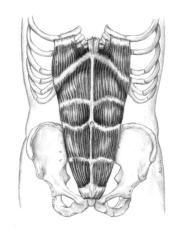

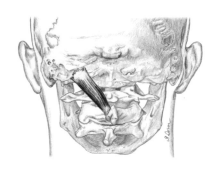

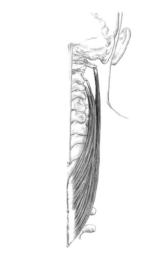

1) _____

2) _____

3) _____

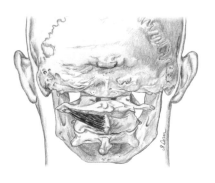

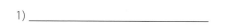

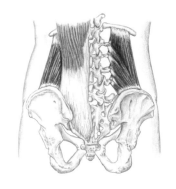

4) _____

5) _____

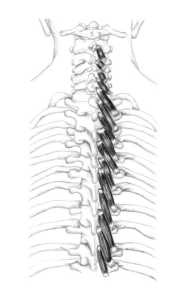

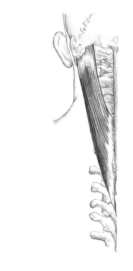

7) _____

6) _____

8) _____

100

Please identify the following muscles.

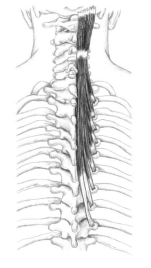

1) _____

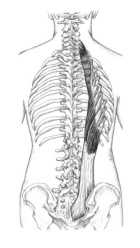

2) _____

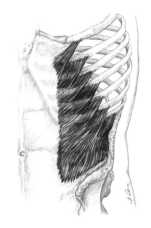

3) _____

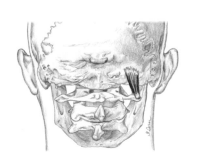

5) _____

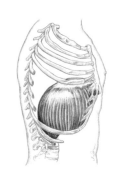

6) _____

4) _____

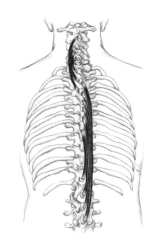

7) _____

8) _____

Please answer the following questions.

1) The most medial branch of the erector spinae group is the _____, while the most

   lateral is the _____.

2) In the lumbar region, the erectors lie deep to what connective tissue structure? _____

3) To contract the lower fibers of the erector spinae group in a prone position, you could ask your partner to perform what action?

   _____

4) When exploring between the scapulae, can you name two muscles through which you will have to palpate to access the deeper erector spinae fibers?

   _____   _____

5) Unlike the long, vertical erector fibers, the branches of the transversospinalis group consist of many

   _____ fibers.

6) As a group, the transversospinalis muscles can be easily located along the _____
   of the thoracic and lumbar vertebrae.

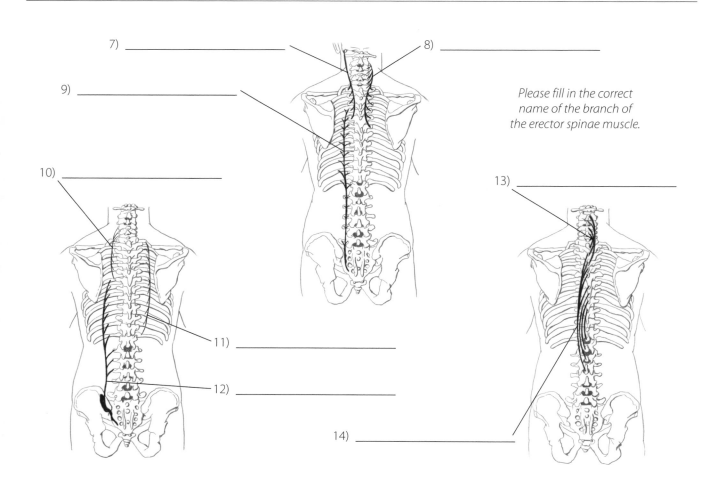

7) _____   8) _____

9) _____

Please fill in the correct name of the branch of the erector spinae muscle.

10) _____   13) _____

11) _____

12) _____

14) _____

Matching

Match the origin and insertion to the correct muscle.

Origins

1) Common tendon (lumborum), posterior surface of ribs 1-12 (thoracis and cervicis)

2) Common tendon (thoracis), TVPs of upper five thoracic vertebrae (cervicis and capitis)

3) Sacrum and TVPs of lumbar through cervical vertebrae

4) Spinous processes of the upper lumbar and lower thoracic vertebrae (thoracis), ligamentum nuchae, spinous process of C-7 (cervicis)

5) TVPs of lumbar through cervical vertebrae

6) TVPs of thoracic vertebrae, articular processes of lower cervicals

Muscle	O	I
Iliocostalis	_____	_____
Longissimus	_____	_____
Multifidi	_____	_____
Rotatores	_____	_____
Semispinalis capitis	_____	_____
Spinalis	_____	_____

Insertions

7) Lower 9 ribs and TVPs of thoracic vertebrae (thoracis), TVPs of cervical vertebrae (cervicis), mastoid process (capitis)

8) Spinous processes of lumbar vertebrae through second cervical vertebra (each belly spanning 1-2 vertebrae)

9) Spinous processes of lumbar vertebrae through second cervical vertebra (each belly spanning 2-4 vertebrae)

10) Spinous processes of upper thoracic (thoracis), spinous processes of cervicals, except C-1 (cervicis)

11) Spinous processes of upper thoracic and cervicals (except C-1), and superior nuchal line of occiput

12) TVPs of lumbar vertebrae 1-3 and posterior surface of ribs 6-12 (lumborum), posterior surface of ribs 1-6 (thoracis), TVPs of lower cervicals (cervicis)

Shorten or Lengthen?

13) Passive flexion of the spine would _____ the iliocostalis.

14) Passive rotation of the spine to the opposite side would _____ the rotatores.

15) Passive lateral flexion of the spine to the same side would _____ the longissimus.

16) Passive rotation of the spine to the same side would _____ the multifidi.

Let's Palpate!

Remember - there are no right or wrong answers here

Locate and explore the **erector spinae group** on three individuals. Then write three words that describe what you feel. (See p. 202-205 in *Trail Guide*)

Person #1 _____

_____

_____

_____

Person #2 _____

_____

_____

_____

Person #3 _____

_____

_____

_____

Please answer the following questions.

1) Rotating the head to the left demands the contraction of which splenius capitis - the left or right?

   _____

2) The splenius capitis is a deep muscle except on the lateral side of the neck where it is superficial between which two muscles?

   _____   _____

3) To distinguish the trapezius fibers from the splenius capitis fibers, you could ask your partner to perform what action?

   _____

4) How can the upper fibers of the trapezius be helpful in locating the suboccipitals?

   _____

5) What two bony landmarks and one region can be helpful to isolate the location of the suboccipitals?

   _____   _____   _____

Please draw the four suboccipital muscles reflecting their correct origins and insertions.

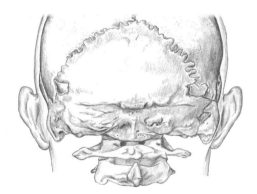

Rectus capitis posterior major

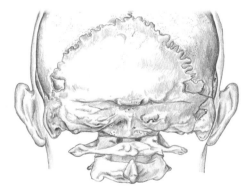

Oblique capitis superior

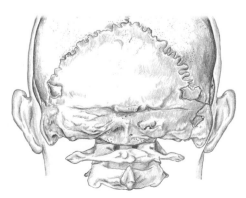

Rectus capitis posterior minor

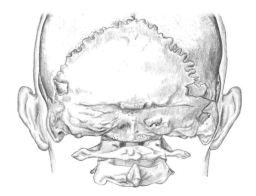

Oblique capitis inferior

Matching

Match the origin and insertion to the correct muscle.

Origins

1) Ligamentum nuchae, spinous processes of C-7 to T-3

2) Spinous process of the axis (C-2) (2)

3) Spinous processes of T-3 to T-6

4) Transverse process of the atlas (C-1)

5) Tubercle of the posterior arch of the atlas (C-1)

Insertions

6) Between the nuchal lines of the occiput

7) Inferior nuchal line of the occiput (2)

8) Mastoid process and lateral portion of superior nuchal line

9) Transverse process of the atlas (C-1)

10) Transverse processes of the upper cervical vertebrae

Muscle	O	I
Oblique capitis inferior	_____	_____
Oblique capitis superior	_____	_____
Rectus capitis posterior major	_____	_____
Rectus capitis posterior minor	_____	_____
Splenius capitis	_____	_____
Splenius cervicis	_____	_____

Let's Palpate!

Remember - there are no right or wrong answers here

Locate and explore the **splenius capitis** on three individuals. Then write three words that describe what you feel.
(See p. 209-210 in *Trail Guide*)

Person #1 _____   Person #2 _____   Person #3 _____

_____   _____   _____

_____   _____   _____

_____   _____   _____

Shorten or Lengthen?

11) Passive rotation of the head to the same side would _____ the rectus capitis posterior major.

12) Passive lateral flexion of the head and neck would _____ the splenius cervicis.

13) Passive extension of the head and neck would _____ the splenius capitis.

14) Passive rotation of the head to the opposite side would _____ the oblique capitis inferior.

15) Passive rotation of the head and neck to the opposite side would _____ the splenius capitis.

QL, Abdominals, Diaphragm and Intercostals

Please answer the following questions.

1) Which edge of the quadratus lumborum is accessible from the side of the torso? _____

2) Which three bony landmarks can help you to isolate the borders of the quadratus lumborum?

_____   _____   _____

3) What action could you ask your partner to perform to feel the quadratus lumborum contract?

_____

4) Which abdominal muscle runs vertically from the rib cage to the pubic crest? _____

5) Rotating your trunk to the right would engage your left or right internal oblique muscle? _____

6) You are palpating lateral to the edge of rectus abdominis and the fibers you feel are superficial and running at an

angle. Which muscle is this? _____

7) What is the primary muscle of respiration? _____

8) When the diaphragm muscle fibers contract, what connective tissue structure is pulled inferiorly?

_____

9) When is it best to move your fingers as you curl them underneath the rib cage to feel the diaphragm?

_____

10) Name two large muscles through which you would have to palpate to access various portions of the intercostals.

_____   _____

Please identify the following structures.

11) _____

12) _____

13) _____

14) _____

15) _____

16) _____

17) _____

18) _____

Color It!

Matching

Match the origin and insertion to the correct muscle.

Origins

1) Inner surface of lower six ribs, upper two or three lumbar vertebrae, inner part of xiphoid process

2) Lateral inguinal ligament, iliac crest and thoracolumbar fascia

3) Lateral inguinal ligament, iliac crest, thoracolumbar fascia and internal surface of lower six ribs

4) Lower eight ribs

5) Posterior iliac crest

6) Pubic crest, pubic symphysis

Insertions

7) Abdominal aponeurosis to linea alba

8) Anterior part of the iliac crest, abdominal aponeurosis to linea alba

9) Cartilage of fifth, sixth and seventh ribs and xiphoid process

10) Central tendon

11) Internal surface of lower three ribs, abdominal aponeurosis to linea alba

12) Last rib and transverse processes of first through fourth lumbar vertebrae

Muscle	O	I
Diaphragm	_____	_____
External oblique	_____	_____
Internal oblique	_____	_____
Quadratus lumborum	_____	_____
Rectus abdominis	_____	_____
Transverse abdominis	_____	_____

Shorten or Lengthen?

13) Increasing the volume of the thoracic cavity would _____ the diaphragm's fibers.

14) Passive rotation of the vertebral column to the same side would _____ the external oblique.

15) Compression of the abdominal contents would _____ the transverse abdominis.

16) Drawing the ventral part of the ribs upward would _____ the external intercostals.

17) Passive rotation of the vertebral column to the opposite side would _____ the internal oblique.

Please answer the following questions.

1) The ligamentum nuchae spans between which two bony landmarks?

_____   _____

2) To feel the ligamentum nuchae change tension underneath your fingers, what two passive movements can you

perform at the head? _____

3) What superficial ligament can be felt between the spinous processes of the thoracic and lumbar vertebrae?

_____

4) The abdominal aorta is located where in relationship to the psoas major? _____

5) The thoracolumbar aponeurosis serves as an attachment site for which two muscles?

_____   _____

Let's Palpate!

Remember - there are no right or wrong answers here

Locate and explore the **quadratus lumborum** on three individuals. Then write three words that describe what you feel.
(See p. 213-214 in *Trail Guide*)

Person #1 _____   Person #2 _____   Person #3 _____

_____   _____   _____

_____   _____   _____

_____   _____   _____

Please identify the following structures.

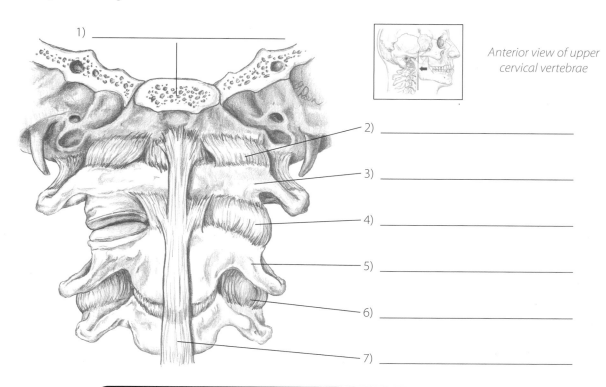

Anterior view of upper cervical vertebrae

1) _____

2) _____

3) _____

4) _____

5) _____

6) _____

7) _____

Color Them!

> ### CHOICES
>
> Alar ligaments
> Anterior longitudinal ligament
> Atlas (2)
> Axis (2)
> Basilar portion of occiput
> Capsule of atlantooccipital joint
>
> Capsule of lateral atlantoaxial joint
> Capsule of zygapophyseal (lateral) joint
> Cruciform ligament
> Inferior longitudinal fibers
> Superior longitudinal fibers
> Transverse ligament of atlas

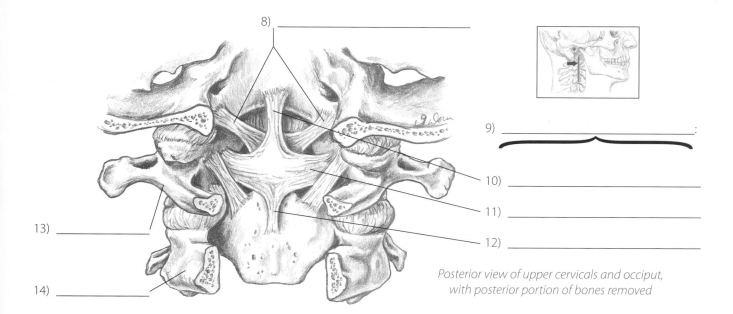

8) _____

9) _____

10) _____

11) _____

12) _____

13) _____

14) _____

Posterior view of upper cervicals and occiput, with posterior portion of bones removed

Please identify the following structures.

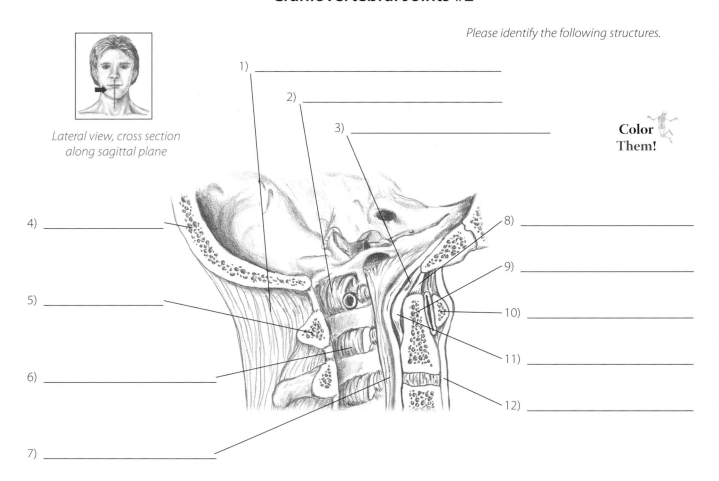

Lateral view, cross section along sagittal plane

Color Them!

1) _____

2) _____

3) _____

4) _____

5) _____

6) _____

7) _____

8) _____

9) _____

10) _____

11) _____

12) _____

CHOICES

Alar ligament
Anterior longitudinal ligament
Anterior tubercle of atlas
Apical ligament
Atlas (2)
Ligamentum nuchae
Occiput
Odontoid process of axis (2)
Posterior atlantoaxial membrane
Posterior atlantooccipital membrane
Posterior longitudinal ligament
Superior longitudinal fibers
   of cruciform ligament
Synovial cavities
Transverse ligament of atlas (2)

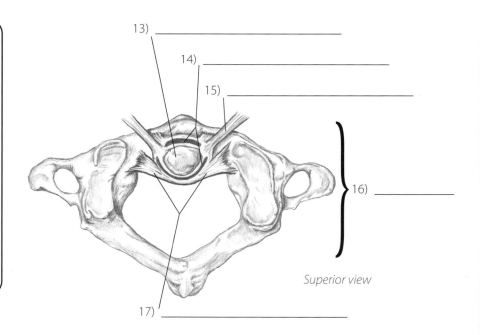

13) _____

14) _____

15) _____

16) _____

17) _____

Superior view

Please identify the following structures.

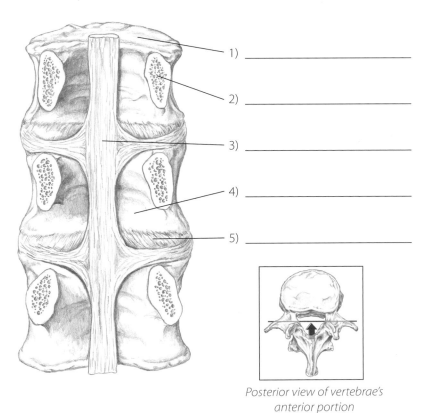

1) _____

2) _____

3) _____

4) _____

5) _____

Posterior view of vertebrae's anterior portion

CHOICES

Body of vertebra
Inferior articular facet
Intervertebral disc
Lamina
Ligamentum flavum
Pedicle (cut) (2)
Posterior longitudinal ligament
Posterior surface of vertebral body
Superior articular process
Transverse process

Color Them!

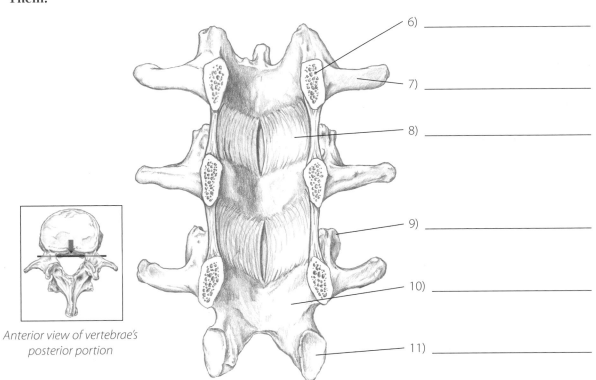

6) _____

7) _____

8) _____

9) _____

10) _____

11) _____

Anterior view of vertebrae's posterior portion

Please identify the following structures.

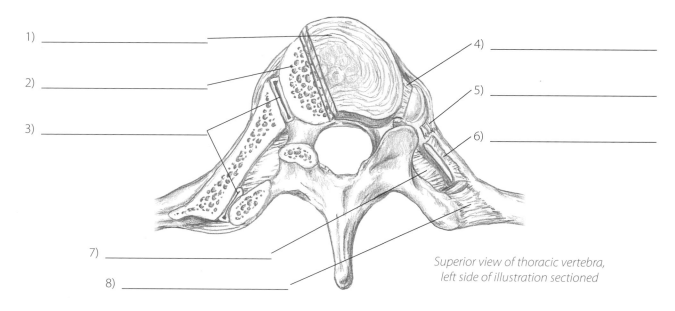

1) _____

2) _____

3) _____

4) _____

5) _____

6) _____

7) _____

8) _____

*Superior view of thoracic vertebra,
left side of illustration sectioned*

CHOICES

Anterior longitudinal ligament	Intervertebral foramen	Spinous process
Body of vertebra (2)	Lateral costotransverse ligament	Superior costotransverse ligament (cut)
Costotransverse ligament	Ligamentum flavum	Supraspinous ligament
Interarticular ligament	Posterior longitudinal ligament	Synovial cavities
Interspinous ligament	Radiate ligament	Transverse process
Intervertebral disc (2)		

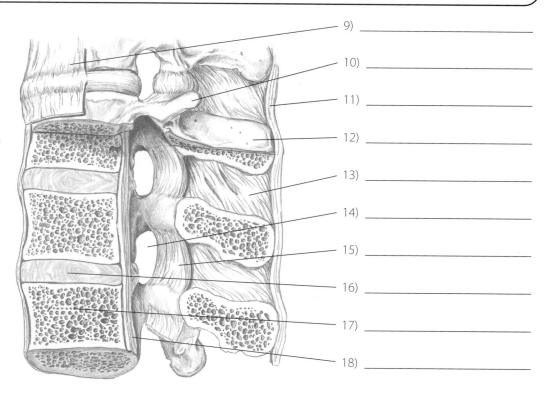

*Lateral view,
partially sectioned*

 **Color
Them!**

9) _____

10) _____

11) _____

12) _____

13) _____

14) _____

15) _____

16) _____

17) _____

18) _____

Please identify the following structures.

1) _____

2) _____

3) _____

4) _____

5) _____

6) _____

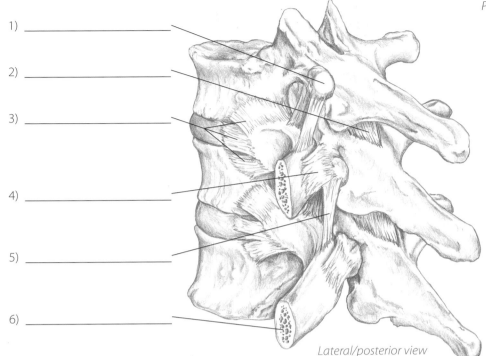

Lateral/posterior view

CHOICES

Articular disc
Clavicle
Costal cartilages
Costoclavicular ligament
Costoxiphoid ligament
Interclavicular ligament
Lateral costotransverse
    ligament
Ligamentum flavum
Radiate ligaments (2)
Rib (cut)
Ribs
Sternocostal joints
Sternomanubrial joint
Superior costotransverse
    ligament
Transverse process
Xiphoid process

Color Them!

7) _____

8) _____

9) _____

14) _____

10) _____

11) _____

15) _____

12) _____

13) _____

16) _____

17) _____

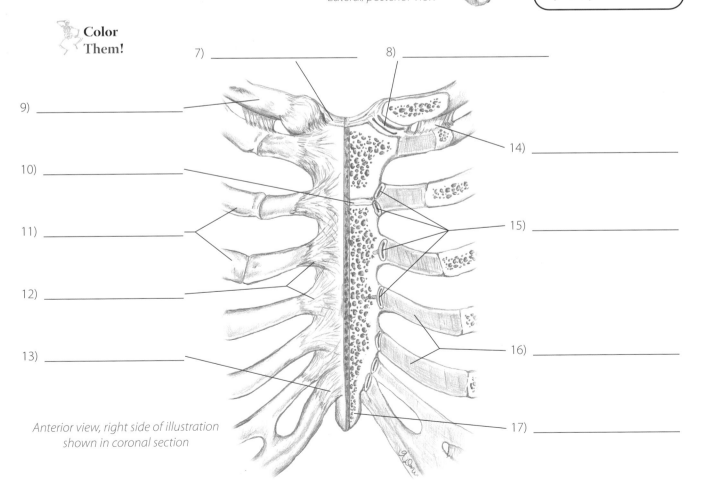

*Anterior view, right side of illustration
shown in coronal section*

Notes

Please identify the following structures.

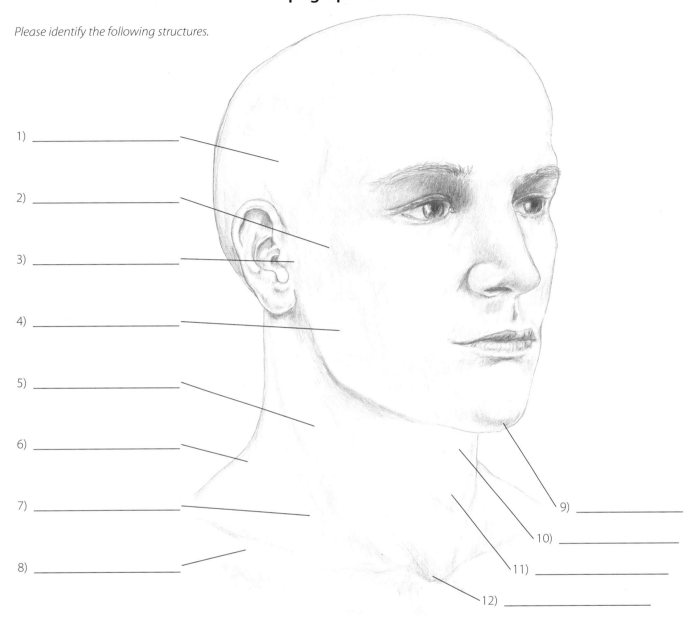

1) _____

2) _____

3) _____

4) _____

5) _____

6) _____

7) _____

8) _____

9) _____

10) _____

11) _____

12) _____

CHOICES

Base of the mandible
Clavicle
Condyle of the mandible
Edge of trapezius
Hyoid bone
Jugular notch
Masseter
Scalenes
Sternocleidomastoid
Temporalis
Thyroid cartilage
Zygomatic arch

Please answer the following questions.

1) What three landmarks create the borders of the neck's anterior triangle? _____

   _____   _____

2) The sternocleidomastoid, clavicle and trapezius form the _____ of the neck.

3) How many bones compose the skull? _____

4) The cranial bones are connected by _____ joints which form tight-fitting sutures.

5) The _____ is located at the posterior and inferior aspects of the cranium.

6) Located at the center of the occiput, the _____ is the superior attachment
   site for the ligamentum nuchae.

7) Which bony landmark of the occiput serves as an attachment site for several neck muscles?

   _____

8) The _____ bones merge at the body's midline to form the sagittal suture.

9) Which bony landmark is located directly behind the earlobe and serves as an attachment site for

   the sternocleidomastoid? _____

10) The space between the zygomatic arch and the cranium is filled by the _____ muscle.

11) The _____ bone forms the forehead and upper rim of the eye sockets.

12) Which bony landmark is located on the underside of the mandible and acts as an attachment site for the

   suprahyoid muscles? _____

13) While palpating the mandible, in which area should one use extra sensitivity? _____

Let's Palpate! _____   *Remember - there are no right or wrong answers here*

Locate and explore the **external occipital protuberance and superior nuchal lines** on three individuals. Then write
three words that describe what you feel. (See p. 237-238 in *Trail Guide*)

Person #1 _____   Person #2 _____   Person #3 _____

_____   _____   _____

_____   _____   _____

_____   _____   _____

Please identify the following structures.

1) _____

2) _____

3) _____

4) _____

5) _____

6) _____

7) _____

8) _____

9) _____

10) _____

11) _____

CHOICES

Ethmoid
External occipital
　　protuberance
Frontal
Lacrimal
Lambdoid suture
Mandible (2)
Mastoid process
Maxilla (2)
Nasal
Occiput
Parietal (2)
Sagittal suture
Sphenoid
Superior nuchal line
Temporal
Vomer
Zygomatic

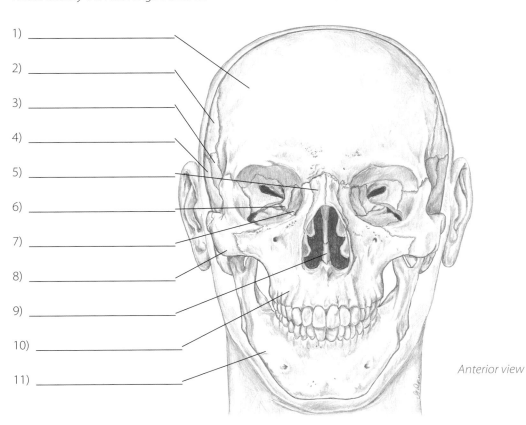

Anterior view

**Color
Them!**

12) _____

13) _____

14) _____

15) _____

16) _____

17) _____

18) _____

19) _____

20) _____

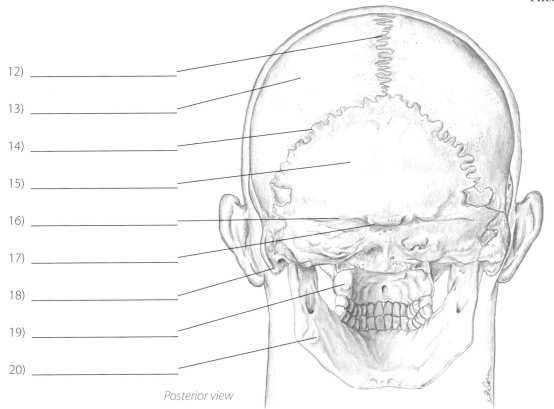

Posterior view

Please identify the following structures. Numbers in bold indicate bones, all others are bony landmarks.

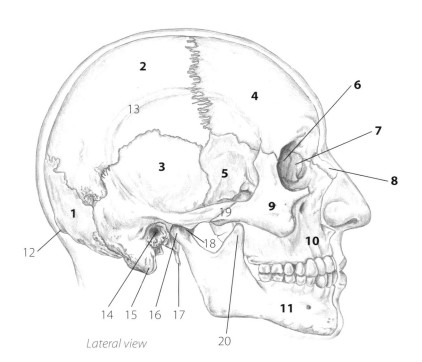

Lateral view

CHOICES 1-20

_____ Condyle of the mandible
_____ Coronoid process
_____ Ethmoid
_____ External auditory meatus
_____ External occipital protuberance
_____ Frontal
_____ Lacrimal
_____ Mandible
_____ Mastoid process
_____ Maxilla
_____ Nasal
_____ Occiput
_____ Parietal
_____ Sphenoid
_____ Styloid process
_____ Temporal
_____ Temporal lines
_____ Temporomandibular joint
_____ Zygomatic
_____ Zygomatic arch

Color Them!

CHOICES 21-32

_____ External occipital protuberance
_____ Foramen magnum
_____ Inferior nuchal line
_____ Mastoid process
_____ Maxilla
_____ Occiput
_____ Palatine
_____ Sphenoid
_____ Superior nuchal line
_____ Temporal
_____ Vomer
_____ Zygomatic

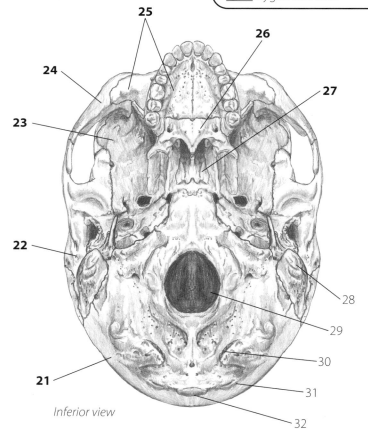

Inferior view

118

Please identify the following structures.

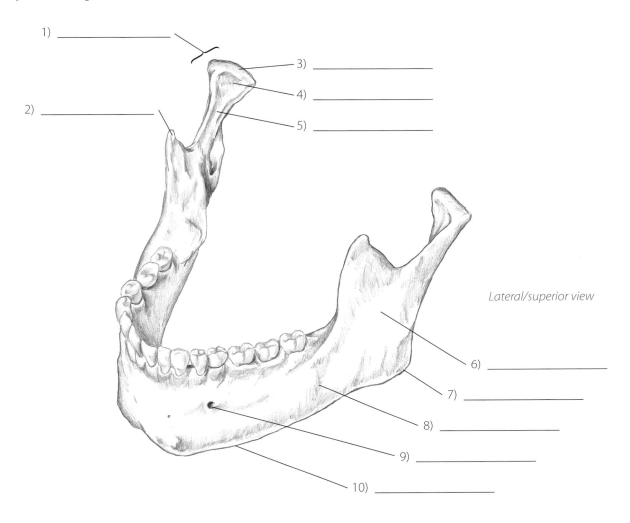

1) _____

2) _____

3) _____

4) _____

5) _____

Lateral/superior view

6) _____

7) _____

8) _____

9) _____

10) _____

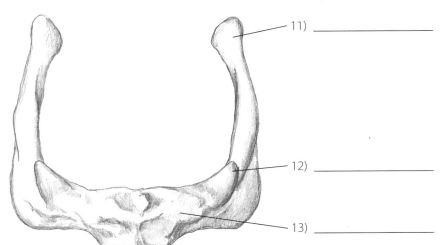

11) _____

12) _____

13) _____

Superior view

CHOICES
Angle
Base
Body (2)
Condyle
Coronoid process
Greater horn
Head
Lesser horn
Mental foramen
Neck
Pterygoid fossa
Ramus

Please identify the following structures.

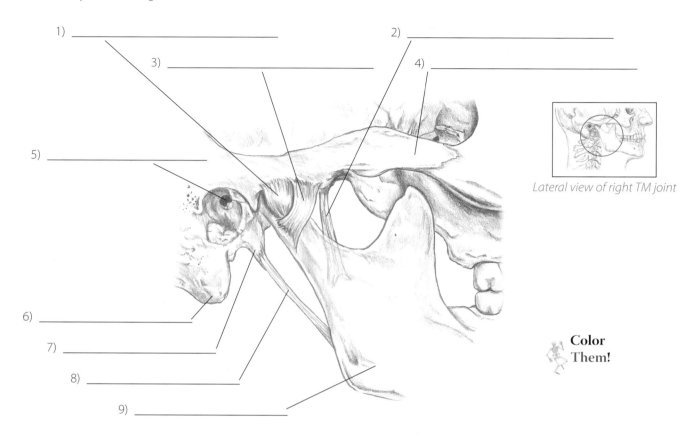

1) _____

3) _____

2) _____

4) _____

Lateral view of right TM joint

5) _____

6) _____

7) _____

8) _____

9) _____

Color Them!

CHOICES

Articular disc of
    temporomandibular joint
Condyle of mandible (cut)
External auditory meatus
Joint capsule (2)
Lateral pterygoid
Lateral temporomandibular
    ligament
Mandible (2)
Mastoid process
Sphenomandibular ligament (2)
Styloid process
Stylomandibular ligament
Zygomatic arch

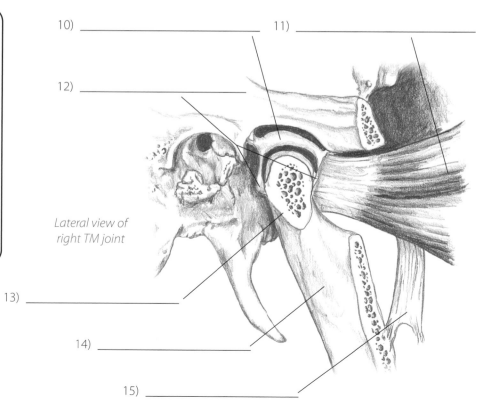

10) _____

11) _____

12) _____

*Lateral view of
right TM joint*

13) _____

14) _____

15) _____

Please identify the following structures.

1) _____

2) _____

3) _____

4) _____

5) _____

6) _____

7) _____

8) _____

9) _____

10) _____

11) _____

12) _____

13) _____

14) _____

15) _____

16) _____

17) _____

18) _____

19) _____

20) _____

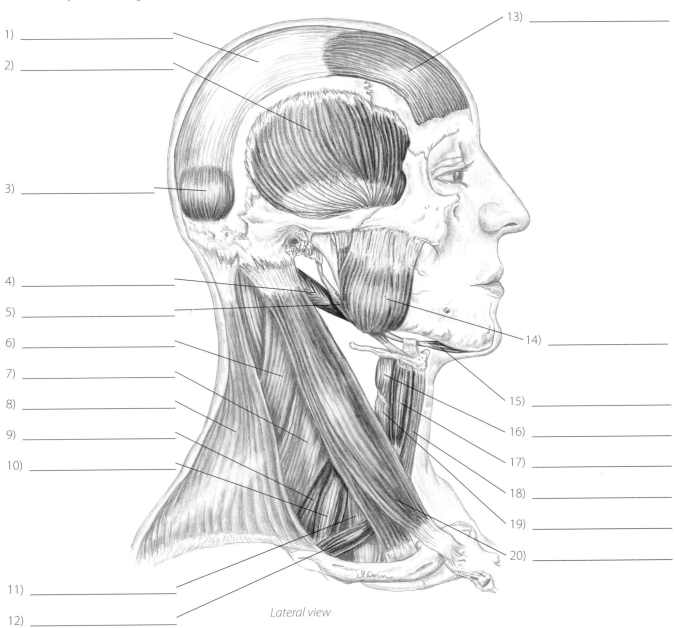

Lateral view

CHOICES

Anterior scalene	Middle scalene	Sternohyoid
Digastric (anterior belly)	Occipitalis	Sternothyroid
Digastric (posterior belly)	Omohyoid (inferior belly)	Stylohyoid
Frontalis	Omohyoid (superior belly)	Temporalis
Galea aponeurotica	Posterior scalene	Thyrohyoid
Levator scapula	Splenius capitis	Trapezius
Masseter	Sternocleidomastoid	

Please identify the following structures.

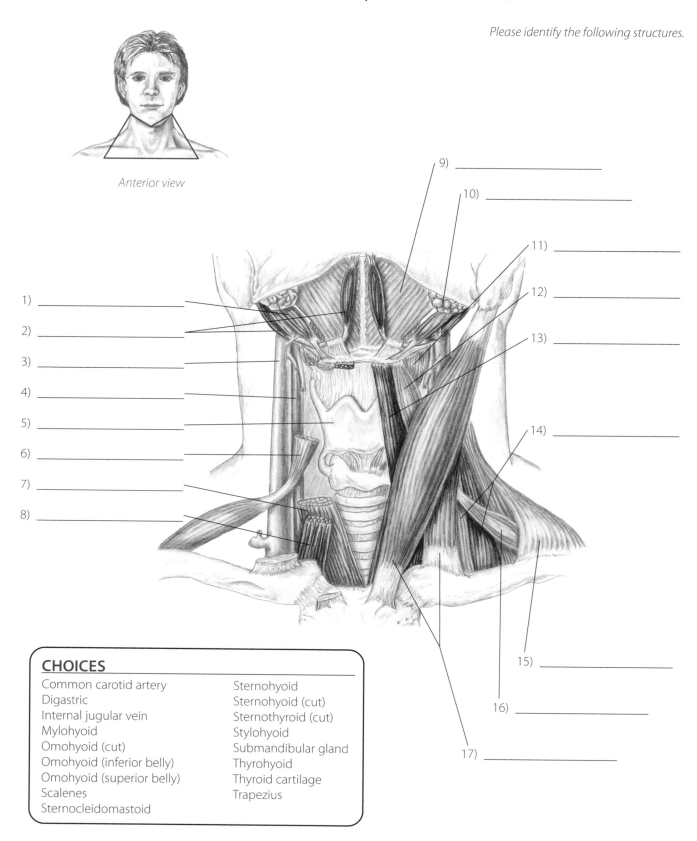

Anterior view

1) _____

2) _____

3) _____

4) _____

5) _____

6) _____

7) _____

8) _____

9) _____

10) _____

11) _____

12) _____

13) _____

14) _____

15) _____

16) _____

17) _____

CHOICES

Common carotid artery
Digastric
Internal jugular vein
Mylohyoid
Omohyoid (cut)
Omohyoid (inferior belly)
Omohyoid (superior belly)
Scalenes
Sternocleidomastoid

Sternohyoid
Sternohyoid (cut)
Sternothyroid (cut)
Stylohyoid
Submandibular gland
Thyrohyoid
Thyroid cartilage
Trapezius

Please identify the following structures.

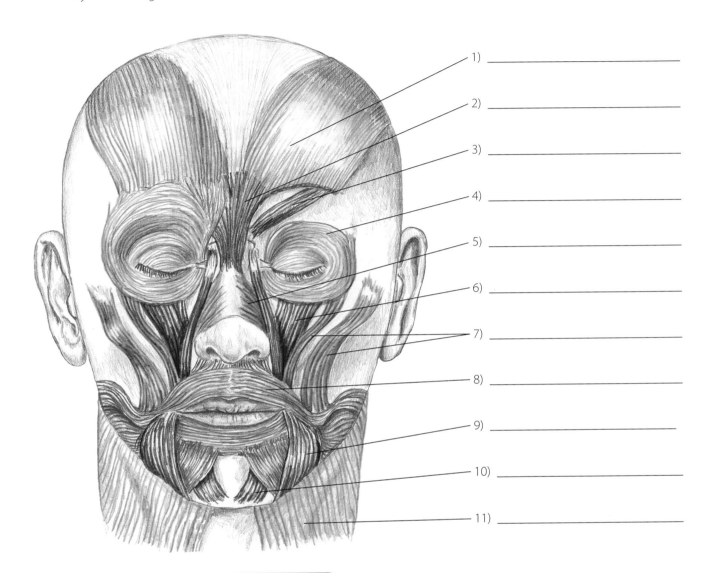

1) _____

2) _____

3) _____

4) _____

5) _____

6) _____

7) _____

8) _____

9) _____

10) _____

11) _____

CHOICES
Corrugator supercili
Depressor anguli oris
Frontalis
Levator labii superioris
Mentalis
Nasalis
Orbicularis oculi
Orbicularis oris
Platysma
Procerus
Zygomaticus major and minor

Using different colors, please fill in and label the muscles and other structures listed below.

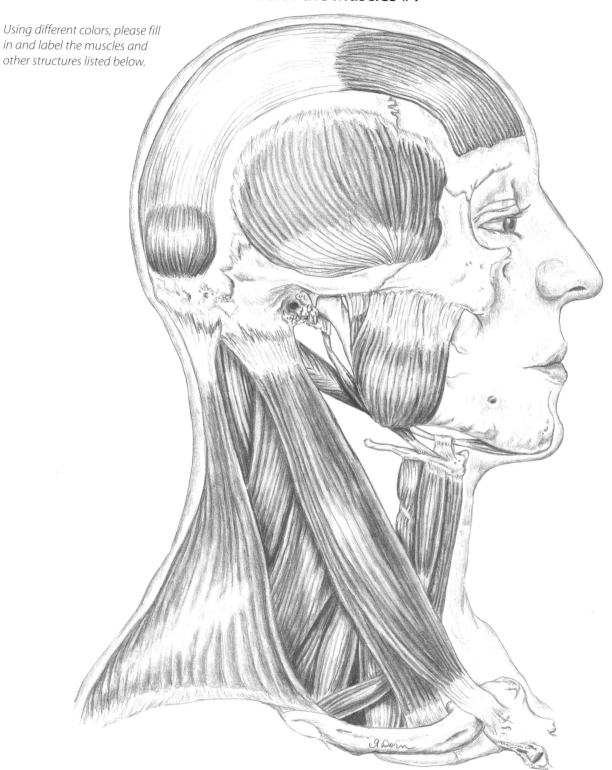

Anterior scalene
Digastric (anterior belly)
Digastric (posterior belly)
Frontalis
Galea aponeurotica

Levator scapula
Masseter
Middle scalene
Occipitalis
Omohyoid (inferior belly)

Omohyoid (superior belly)
Posterior scalene
Splenius capitis
Sternocleidomastoid
Sternohyoid

Sternothyroid
Stylohyoid
Temporalis
Thyrohyoid
Trapezius

Using different colors, please fill in and label the muscles listed below.

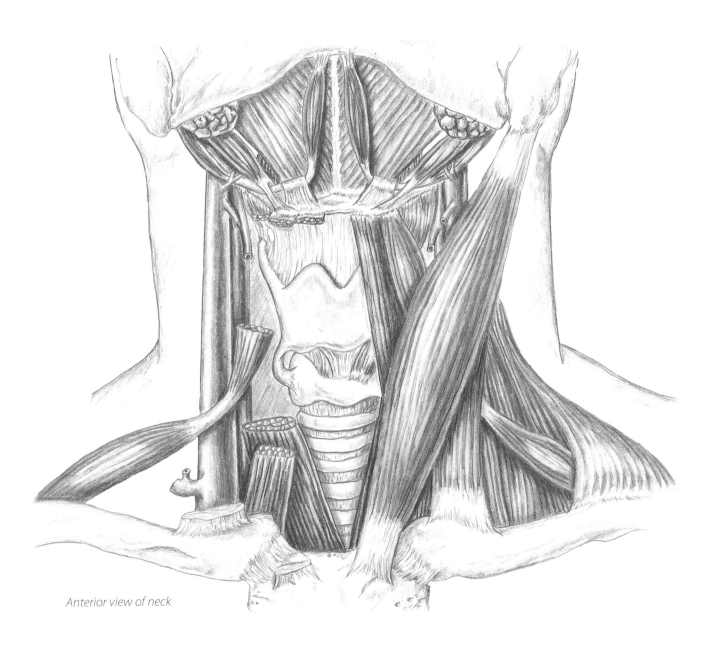

Anterior view of neck

Common carotid artery	Omohyoid (inferior belly)	Sternohyoid	Submandibular gland
Digastric	Omohyoid (superior belly)	Sternohyoid (cut)	Thyrohyoid
Internal jugular vein	Scalenes	Sternothyroid (cut)	Thyroid cartilage
Mylohyoid	Sternocleidomastoid	Stylohyoid	Trapezius
Omohyoid (cut)			

*Using different colors, please fill in and label the
muscles and other structures listed below.*

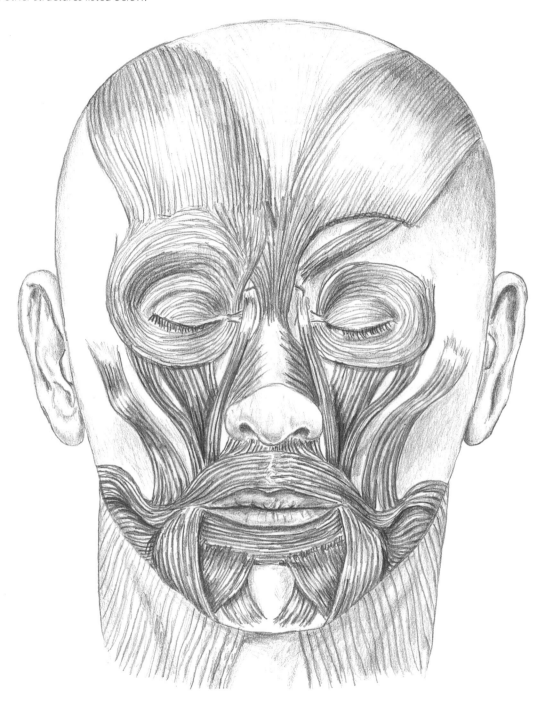

Corrugator supercili	Levator labii superioris	Orbicularis oculi	Procerus
Depressor anguli oris	Mentalis	Orbicularis oris	Zygomaticus
Frontalis	Nasalis	Platysma	major and minor

126

Please list the action demonstrated, synergists and antagonist(s).

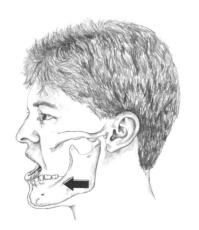

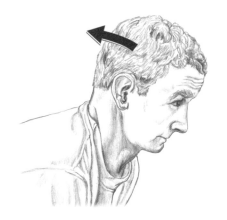

1) Action

_____

2) Synergists

_____

_____

3) Antagonists

_____

_____

4) Action

_____

5) Synergists

S _____

S _____

6) Antagonist

S _____

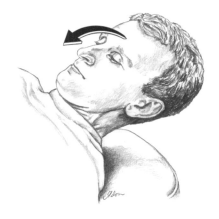

7) Action

_____

8) Synergists

L _____

L _____

9) Antagonist

L _____

Please list the action demonstrated, two synergists and one antagonist.
The first letter of the muscles has been provided.

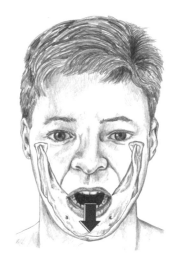

1) Action

_____

2) Synergists

G _____

D _____

3) Antagonist

T _____

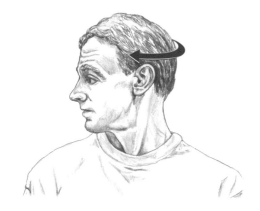

4) Action (to his right)

_____

5) Synergists (and on what side - his left or right?)

M _____

T _____

6) Antagonist (and on what side - his left or right?)

L _____

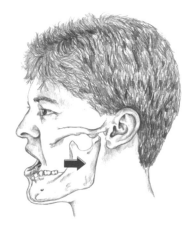

7) Action

_____

8) Synergists

T _____

D _____

9) Antagonist

L _____

Please list the action demonstrated, synergists and antagonist.
The first letter of the muscles has been provided.

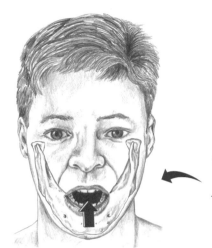

1) This action happens at which joint?

_____

2) Action

_____

3) Synergists

T_____

M_____

4) Antagonist

G_____

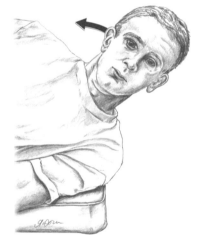

5) Action

_____

6) Synergists

S_____

S_____

S_____

Head, Neck and Face
What's the Muscle? #1

Please identify the following muscles.

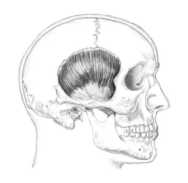

1) _____

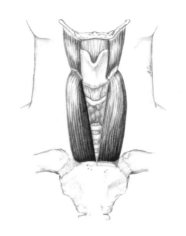

2) _____

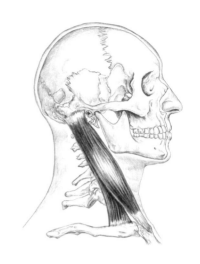

3) _____

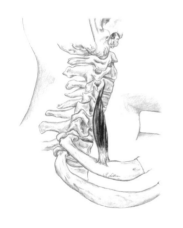

4) _____

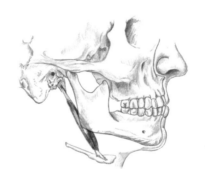

5) _____

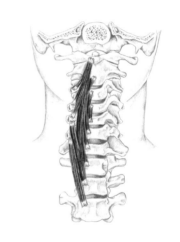

6) _____

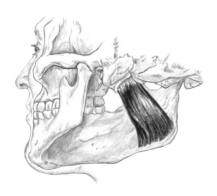

7) _____

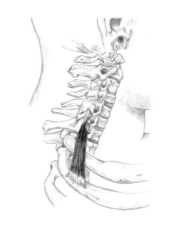

8) _____

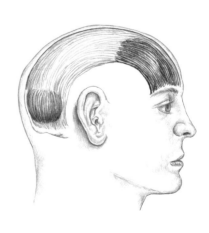

9) _____

130

Please identify the following muscles.

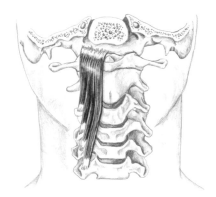

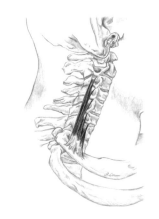

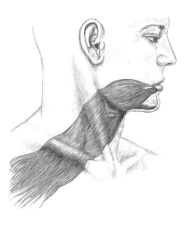

1) _____

2) _____

3) _____

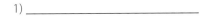
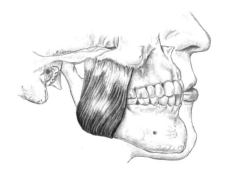

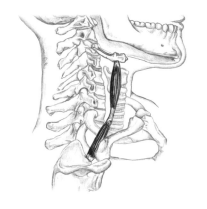

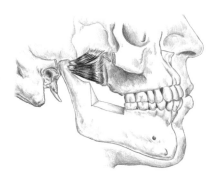

4) _____

5) _____

6) _____

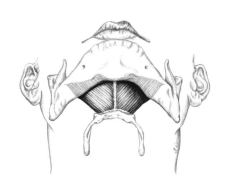

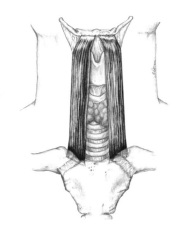

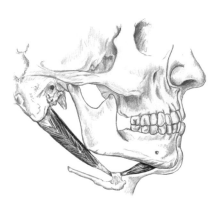

7) _____

8) _____

9) _____

Please answer the following questions.

1) The two heads of the sternocleidomastoid originate at the _____ and the _____.

2) To create an even more visible contraction in the sternocleidomastoid (SCM), ask your partner to flex her neck after

   making what adjustment? _____

3) Which scalene is difficult to distinguish from surrounding muscle bellies? _____

4) Which muscles are located between the SCM and the anterior flap of the trapezius? _____

5) The brachial plexus and subclavian artery pass through a small gap between which two muscles on the
   anterior, lateral neck?

   _____   _____

6) You might ask your partner to "breathe deeply into your upper chest" when palpating which muscle group?

   _____

7) The anterior scalene lies partially deep to the lateral edge of which muscle? _____

8) To discern the posterior scalene from the levator scapula, what action could you ask your partner to perform that

   would contract the levator but not the scalene? _____

9) The _____ is the strongest muscle in the body relative to its size.

10) The broad origin of which muscle attaches to the frontal, temporal and parietal bones? _____

11) To access the insertion of the temporalis, you must ask your partner to perform what action?

   _____

Shorten or Lengthen? _____

12) Passive protraction of the mandible would _____ the temporalis.

13) Passive rotation of the head and neck to the opposite side would _____ the scalenes.

14) Passive lateral flexion of the head and neck to the same side would _____ the sternocleidomastoid
    and scalenes.

15) Passive flexion of the head and neck would _____ the anterior scalene.

16) Passive rotation of the head and neck to the same side would _____ the sternocleidomastoid.

17) Passive elevation of the mandible would _____ the masseter.

Matching

Match the origin and insertion to the correct muscle.

Origins

1) Temporal fossa and fascia

2) Top of manubrium, medial one-third of the clavicle

3) Transverse processes of fifth and sixth cervical vertebrae (posterior tubercles)

4) Transverse processes of second through seventh cervical vertebrae (posterior tubercles)

5) Transverse processes of third through sixth cervical vertebrae (anterior tubercles)

6) Zygomatic arch

Insertions

7) Angle and ramus of mandible

8) Coronoid process of the mandible

9) First rib (2)

10) Mastoid process of temporal bone and the lateral portion of superior nuchal line of occiput

11) Second rib

Muscle	O	I
Anterior scalene	_____	_____
Masseter	_____	_____
Middle scalene	_____	_____
Posterior scalene	_____	_____
Sternocleidomastoid	_____	_____
Temporalis	_____	_____

Let's Palpate!

Remember - there are no right or wrong answers here

Locate and explore the **sternocleidomastoid** on three individuals. Then write three words that describe what you feel. (See p. 250-251 in *Trail Guide*)

Person #1 _____

Person #2 _____

Person #3 _____

_____   _____   _____

_____   _____   _____

_____   _____   _____

Please answer the following questions.

1) Name the four muscles which comprise the suprahyoids.

   _____   _____

   _____   _____

2) Which muscle originates at the mastoid process, loops through a tendinous sling at the hyoid bone and inserts to the inferior border of the mandible? _____

3) What direction should you give your partner in order to locate the suprahyoids? _____

4) Which muscle runs from the hyoid bone to the superior border of the scapula and is mostly inaccessible?

   _____

5) Which muscle becomes visually distinct when your partner forms a *Creature from the Black Lagoon* expression?

   _____

6) The galea aponeurotica forms the bridge between which two muscle bellies?

   _____   _____

7) The frontalis is best seen and felt by asking your partner to do what action?

   _____

8) What two muscles attach from the anterior surface of the cervical vertebrae to the occiput and atlas?

   _____   _____

Let's Palpate!

Remember - there are no right or wrong answers here

Locate and explore the **suprahyoids** on three individuals. Then write three words that describe what you feel.
(See p. 259-260 in *Trail Guide*)

Person #1 _____   Person #2 _____   Person #3 _____

_____   _____   _____

_____   _____   _____

_____   _____   _____

Matching

Match the origin and insertion to the correct muscle.

Origins

1) Top of manubrium (2)

2) Mastoid process

3) Styloid process

4) Superior border of the scapula

5) Underside of mandible (2)

Insertions

6) Hyoid bone (5)

7) Inferior border of the mandible

8) Thyroid cartilage

Muscle	O	I
Digastric	_____	_____
Geniohyoid	_____	_____
Mylohyoid	_____	_____
Omohyoid	_____	_____
Sternohyoid	_____	_____
Sternothyroid	_____	_____
Stylohyoid	_____	_____

Shorten or Lengthen?

9) Passively raising the eyebrows would _____ the frontalis fibers.

10) Tightening the fascia of the neck would _____ the platysma.

11) Passive protraction of the mandible would _____ the digastric.

12) Passive depression of the mandible would _____ the suprahyoids.

13) Not that you'd ever want to, but passive elevation of the hyoid bone would _____ the infrahyoids.

Please identify the following structures.

1) _____

2) _____

3) _____

4) _____

5) _____

6) _____

Color Me!

7) _____

8) _____

9) _____

10) _____

11) _____

12) _____

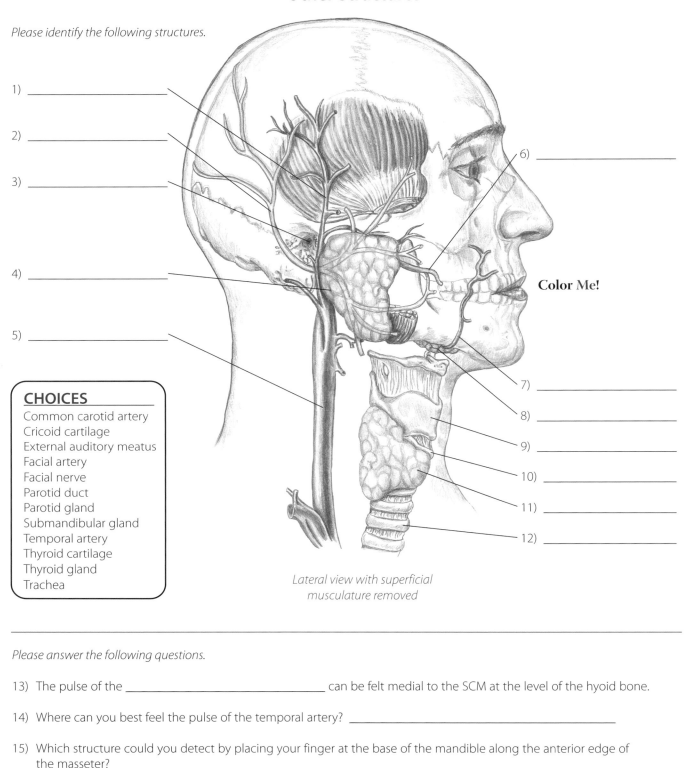

Lateral view with superficial musculature removed

CHOICES

Common carotid artery
Cricoid cartilage
External auditory meatus
Facial artery
Facial nerve
Parotid duct
Parotid gland
Submandibular gland
Temporal artery
Thyroid cartilage
Thyroid gland
Trachea

Please answer the following questions.

13) The pulse of the _____ can be felt medial to the SCM at the level of the hyoid bone.

14) Where can you best feel the pulse of the temporal artery? _____

15) Which structure could you detect by placing your finger at the base of the mandible along the anterior edge of the masseter?

_____

16) The thyroid gland is situated on the anterior surface of the trachea between which two structures?

_____   _____

Please identify the following structures.

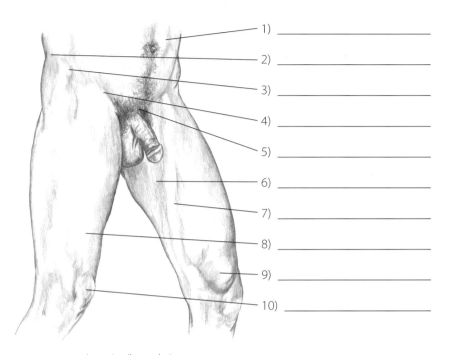

1) _____

2) _____

3) _____

4) _____

5) _____

6) _____

7) _____

8) _____

9) _____

10) _____

Anterior/lateral view

CHOICES

Adductors
Anterior superior iliac spine
Coccyx
Gluteal cleft
Gluteal fold
Gluteus maximus
Gluteus medius
Greater trochanter
Hamstring tendons
Hamstrings
Iliac crest
Iliotibial tract
Inguinal ligament
Patella
Popliteal fossa
Posterior superior iliac spine
Pubic crest
Rectus abdominis
Rectus femoris
Sacrum
Sartorius
Vastus lateralis
Vastus medialis

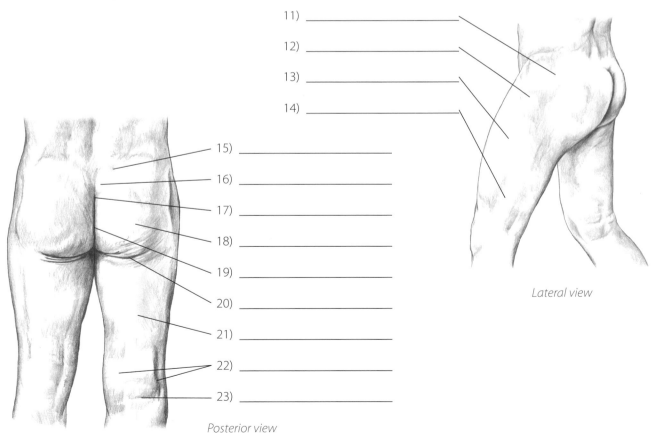

11) _____

12) _____

13) _____

14) _____

15) _____

16) _____

17) _____

18) _____

19) _____

20) _____

21) _____

22) _____

23) _____

Posterior view

Lateral view

Please answer the following questions.

1) Name the three bones which make up the hip (coxal) bone.

   _____   _____   _____

2) The _____ and _____ are considered part of both the pelvis and the vertebral column.

3) Describe the difference between a typical male and female pelvis.

   _____

4) The _____ can be palpated by following the superior pelvis from the ASIS to the PSIS on the side of the torso.

5) Which pair of bony landmarks can be visually identified by two small dimples at the base of the lower back?

   _____

6) The _____ are often called the "sits bones."

7) Which large bony landmark can be located by sliding your fingerpads inferiorly four to six inches along the lateral side of

   the thigh? _____

8) The _____ is located on the medial surface of the ilium and serves as an attachment site for the iliacus muscle.

Let's Palpate!

Remember - there are no right or wrong answers here

Locate and explore the **anterior superior iliac spines (ASISes)** on three individuals. Then write three words that describe what you feel. (See p. 283 in *Trail Guide*)

Person #1 _____   Person #2 _____   Person #3 _____

_____   _____   _____

_____   _____   _____

_____   _____   _____

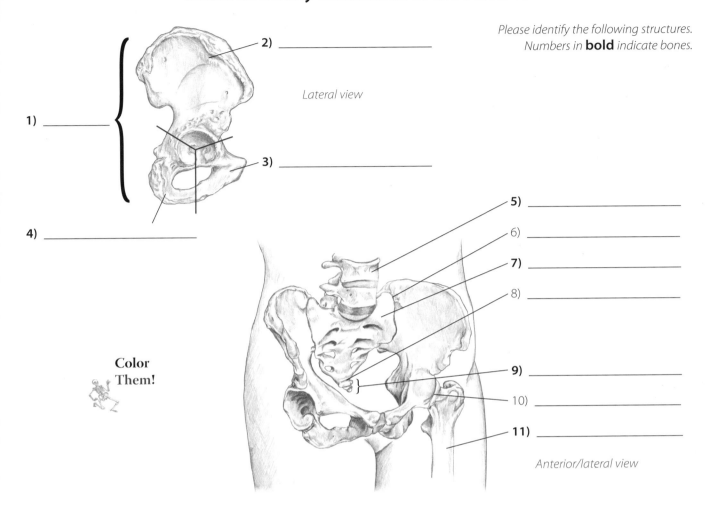

Please identify the following structures.
*Numbers in **bold** indicate bones.*

2) _____

Lateral view

1) _____

3) _____

4) _____

5) _____

6) _____

7) _____

8) _____

Color Them!

9) _____

10) _____

11) _____

Anterior/lateral view

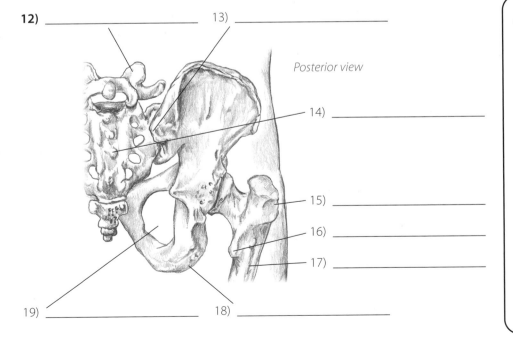

12) _____

13) _____

Posterior view

14) _____

15) _____

16) _____

17) _____

19) _____

18) _____

CHOICES
Coccyx
Coxal (hip) joint
Femur
Fifth lumbar vertebra
Gluteal tuberosity
Greater trochanter
Hip
Ilium
Ischial tuberosity
Ischium
Lesser trochanter
Lumbar vertebra
Medial sacral crest
Obturator foramen
Posterior superior iliac spine (PSIS)
Pubis
Sacrococcygeal joint
Sacroiliac joint
Sacrum

1) _____

2) _____

3) _____

Anterior surface

4) _____

5) _____

6) _____

7) _____

8) _____

9) _____

Please identify the following structures.

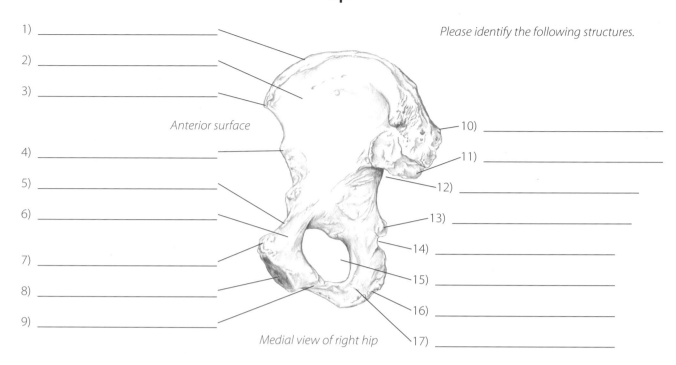

10) _____

11) _____

12) _____

13) _____

14) _____

15) _____

16) _____

17) _____

Medial view of right hip

CHOICES

Acetabulum	Inferior gluteal line	Posterior gluteal line
Anterior gluteal line	Inferior ramus of pubis (2)	Posterior inferior iliac spine (2)
Anterior inferior iliac spine (2)	Ischial spine (2)	Posterior superior iliac spine (2)
Anterior superior iliac spine (2)	Ischial tuberosity (2)	Pubic tubercle (2)
Greater sciatic notch (2)	Lesser sciatic notch (2)	Ramus of the ischium
Iliac crest (2)	Obturator foramen (2)	Superior ramus of pubis (2)
Iliac fossa	Pectineal line	Symphyseal surface
Iliac tubercle		

18) _____

19) _____

20) _____

21) _____

22) _____

23) _____

24) _____

25) _____

26) _____

27) _____

28) _____

29) _____

Anterior surface

30) _____

31) _____

32) _____

33) _____

34) _____

35) _____

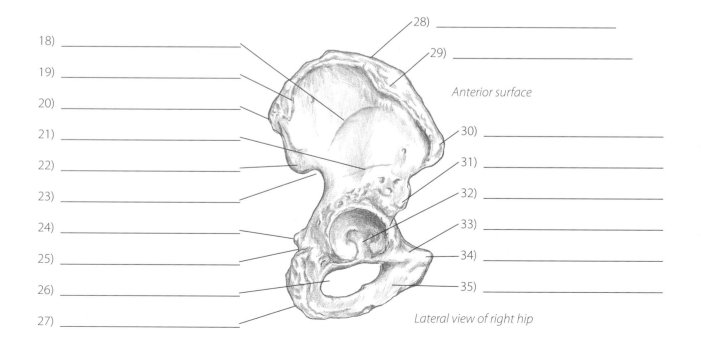

Lateral view of right hip

Please identify the following structures.

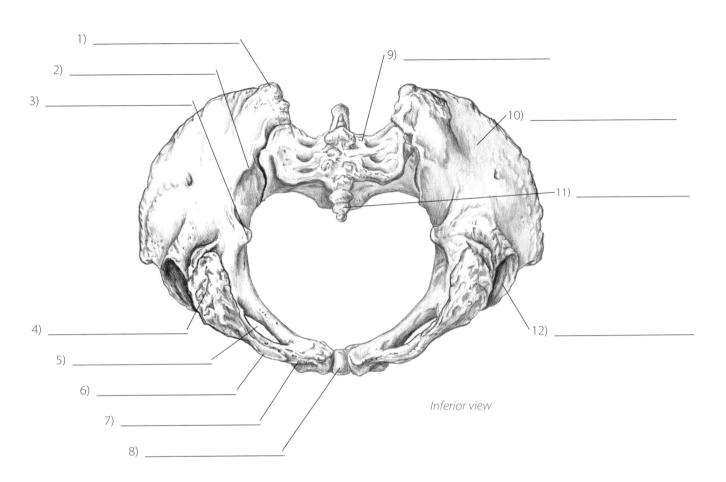

1) _____

2) _____

3) _____

9) _____

10) _____

11) _____

4) _____

5) _____

6) _____

7) _____

8) _____

12) _____

Inferior view

CHOICES
Acetabulum
Coccyx
Gluteal surface of ilium
Inferior ramus of pubis
Ischial spine
Ischial tuberosity
Obturator foramen
Posterior inferior iliac spine
Posterior superior iliac spine
Pubic symphysis
Ramus of ischium
Sacrum

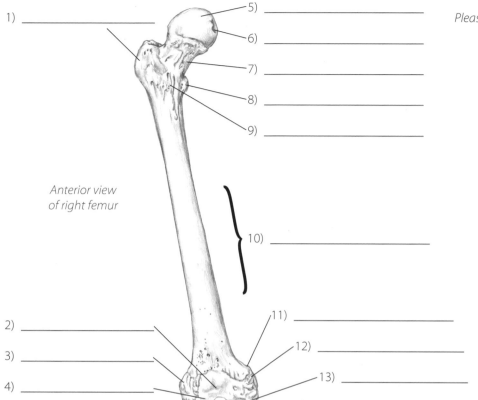

1) _____

2) _____

3) _____

4) _____

*Anterior view
of right femur*

5) _____

6) _____

7) _____

8) _____

9) _____

10) _____

11) _____

12) _____

13) _____

Please identify the following structures.

CHOICES

Adductor tubercle (2)
Fovea of head
Gluteal tuberosity
Greater trochanter (2)
Head (2)
Intercondylar fossa
Intertrochanteric crest
Intertrochanteric line
Lateral condyle (2)
Lateral epicondyle (2)
Lateral lip of linea aspera
Lesser trochanter (2)
Medial condyle (2)
Medial epicondyle (2)
Medial lip of linea aspera
Neck (2)
Patellar surface
Pectineal line
Shaft
Trochanteric fossa

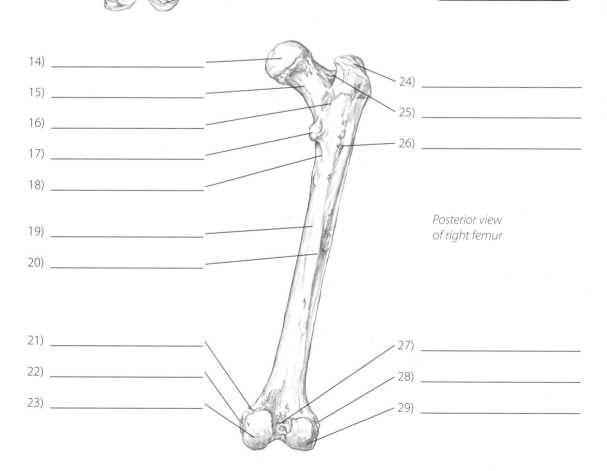

14) _____

15) _____

16) _____

17) _____

18) _____

19) _____

20) _____

21) _____

22) _____

23) _____

24) _____

25) _____

26) _____

*Posterior view
of right femur*

27) _____

28) _____

29) _____

Please answer the following questions.

1) The _____ is comprised of 4-5 fused vertebrae and the _____ is comprised of 3-4 fused bones.

2) The ridge running down the center of the sacrum is the _____.

3) The coccyx is located nearest to which topographical feature? _____

4) The _____ joint can be found just inferior and medial to the PSIS.

5) With your partner prone, what passive positional adjustment and motion will help you to feel movement in the sacroiliac joint?

_____

6) Which bony landmark can be found just distal to the greater trochanter and directly lateral to the ischial tuberosity?

_____

7) What are a couple ways to increase comfort for both you and your partner while palpating in the pubic region?

_____

8) The _____ are the bony prominences located on the superior part of the pubic crest.

9) The superior ramus of the pubis forms a ridge that serves as an attachment site for the _____.

10) The rami of the pubis form a bridge between the _____ and the

_____.

11) What is the recommended position of your partner while palpating the pubic rami?

_____

12) The _____ is the horizontal line between the buttock and thigh.

Let's Palpate!

Remember - there are no right or wrong answers here

Locate and explore the **pubic crest and tubercles** on three individuals. Then write three words that describe what you feel. (See p. 291 and 292 in *Trail Guide*)

Person #1 _____   Person #2 _____   Person #3 _____

_____   _____   _____

_____   _____   _____

_____   _____   _____

Please identify the following structures.

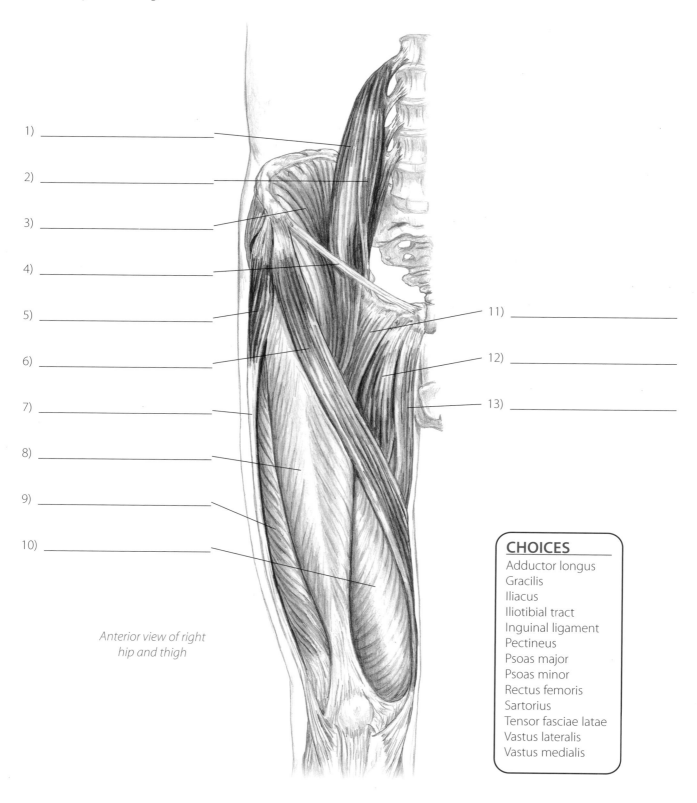

1) _____

2) _____

3) _____

4) _____

5) _____

6) _____

7) _____

8) _____

9) _____

10) _____

11) _____

12) _____

13) _____

*Anterior view of right
hip and thigh*

CHOICES
Adductor longus
Gracilis
Iliacus
Iliotibial tract
Inguinal ligament
Pectineus
Psoas major
Psoas minor
Rectus femoris
Sartorius
Tensor fasciae latae
Vastus lateralis
Vastus medialis

Please identify the following structures.

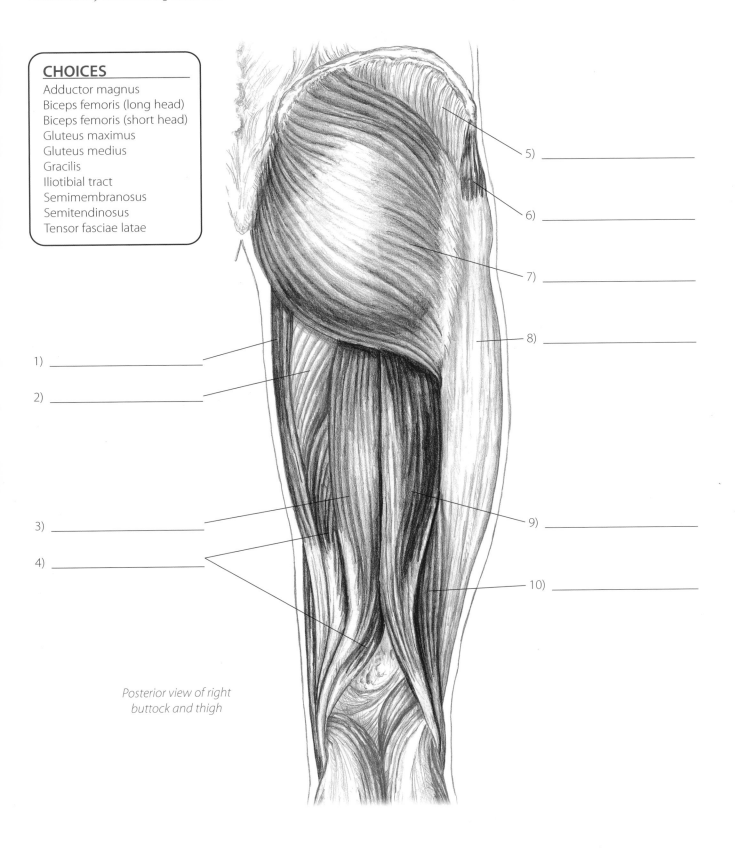

CHOICES
Adductor magnus
Biceps femoris (long head)
Biceps femoris (short head)
Gluteus maximus
Gluteus medius
Gracilis
Iliotibial tract
Semimembranosus
Semitendinosus
Tensor fasciae latae

1) _____

2) _____

3) _____

4) _____

5) _____

6) _____

7) _____

8) _____

9) _____

10) _____

*Posterior view of right
buttock and thigh*

Please identify the following structures.

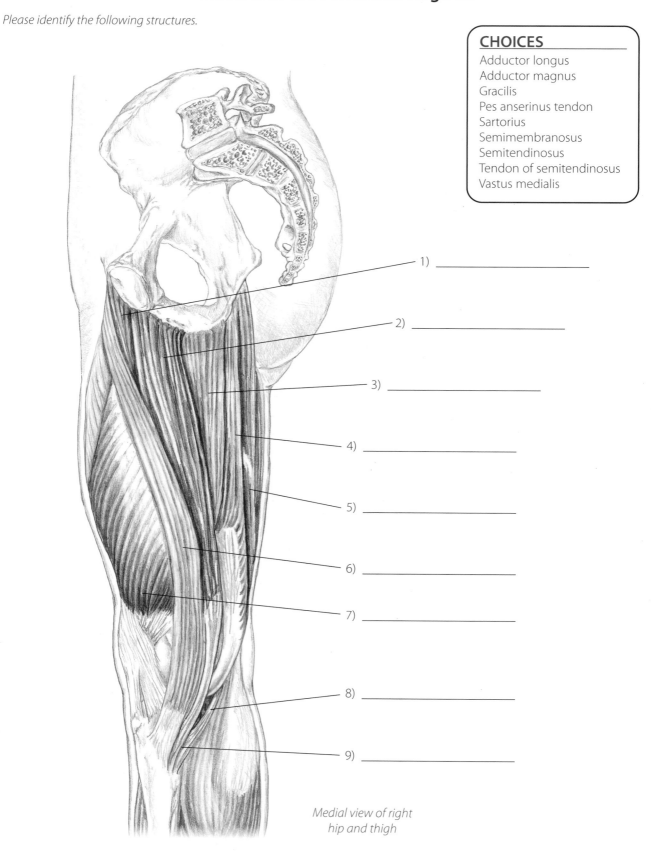

1) _____

2) _____

3) _____

4) _____

5) _____

6) _____

7) _____

8) _____

9) _____

*Medial view of right
hip and thigh*

Please identify the following structures.

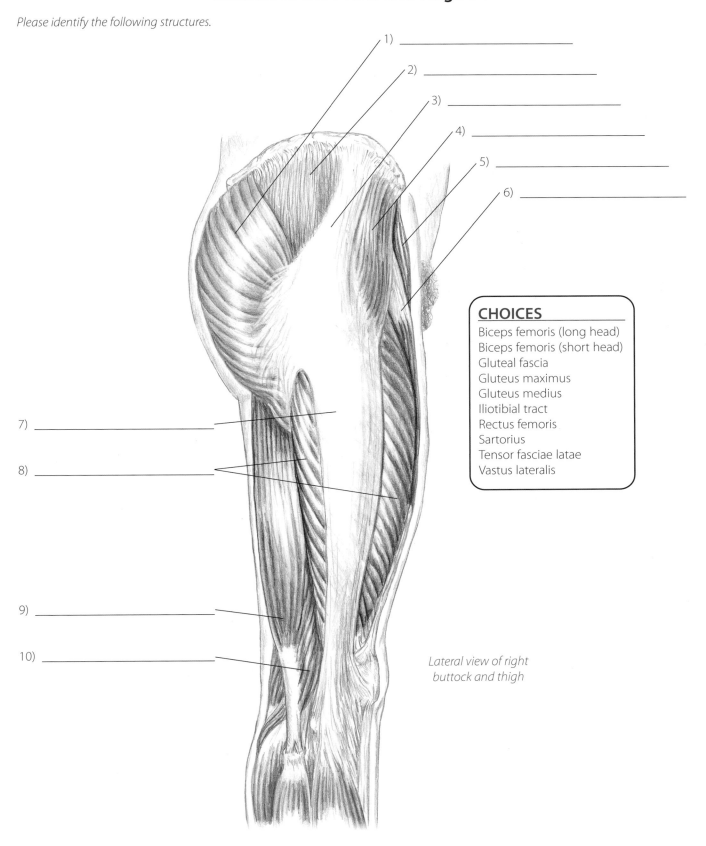

1) _____

2) _____

3) _____

4) _____

5) _____

6) _____

7) _____

8) _____

9) _____

10) _____

CHOICES
Biceps femoris (long head)
Biceps femoris (short head)
Gluteal fascia
Gluteus maximus
Gluteus medius
Iliotibial tract
Rectus femoris
Sartorius
Tensor fasciae latae
Vastus lateralis

Lateral view of right buttock and thigh

*Using different colors, please fill in and label
the muscles and other structures listed below.*

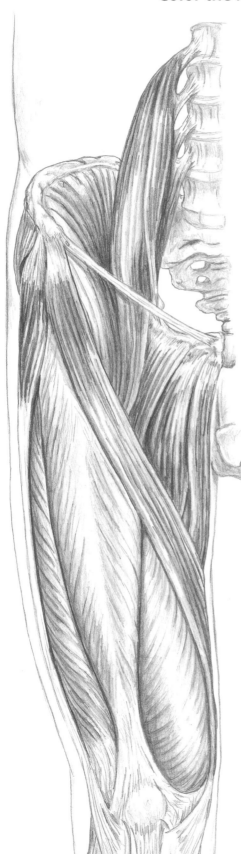

Adductor longus
Gracilis
Iliacus
Iliotibial tract
Inguinal ligament
Pectineus
Psoas major
Psoas minor
Rectus femoris
Sartorius
Tensor fasciae latae
Vastus lateralis
Vastus medialis

*Anterior view of right
hip and thigh*

*Using different colors, please fill in and label
the muscles and other structures listed below.*

Adductor magnus
Biceps femoris (long head)
Biceps femoris (short head)
Gluteus maximus
Gluteus medius
Gracilis
Iliotibial tract
Semimembranosus
Semitendinosus
Tensor fasciae latae

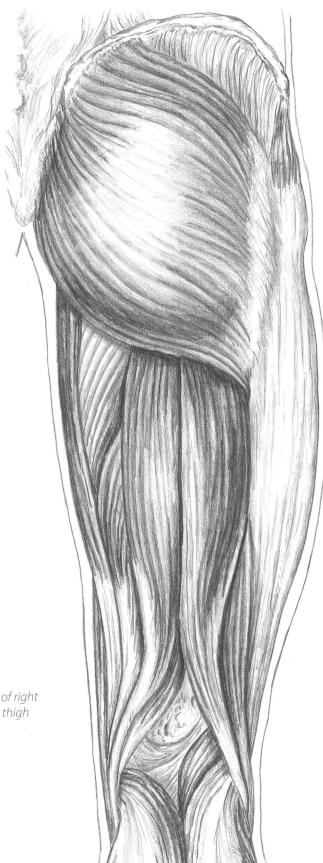

*Posterior view of right
buttock and thigh*

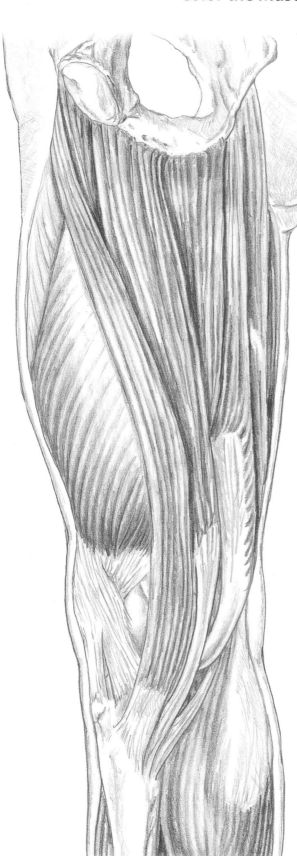

Using different colors, please fill in and label the muscles and other structures listed below.

Adductor longus
Adductor magnus
Gracilis
Pes anserinus tendon
Sartorius
Semimembranosus
Semitendinosus
Tendon of semitendinosus
Vastus medialis

Medial view of right hip and thigh

150

Using different colors, please fill in and label the muscles and other structures listed below.

Biceps femoris (long head)
Biceps femoris (short head)
Gluteal fascia
Gluteus maximus
Gluteus medius
Iliotibial tract
Rectus femoris
Sartorius
Tensor fasciae latae
Vastus lateralis

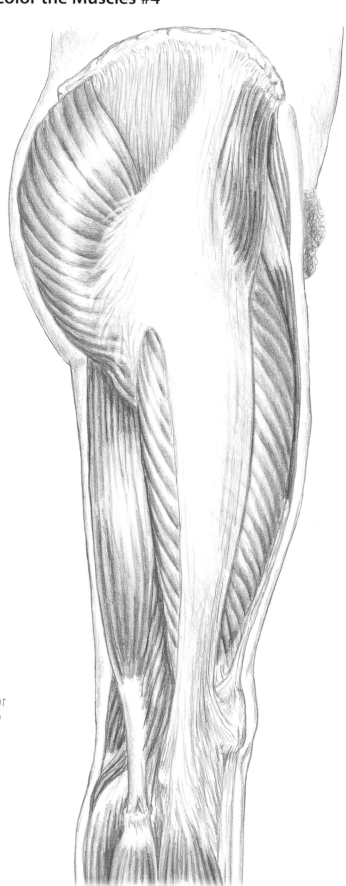

Lateral view of right buttock and thigh

Please list the action demonstrated, two synergists and one antagonist.
The first letter of the muscles has been provided.

1) This action happens at which joint?

_____

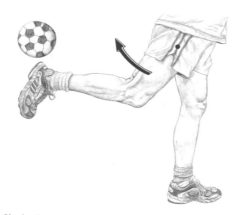

2) Action

_____

3) Synergists

B _____

A _____

4) Antagonist

R _____

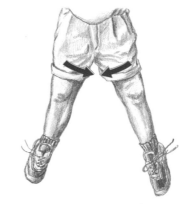

5) Action

_____

6) Synergists

G _____

I _____

7) Antagonist

T _____

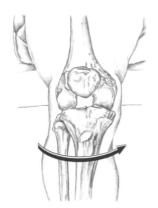

8) Action

_____

9) Synergists

S _____

P _____

10) Antagonist

B _____

Please list the action demonstrated, two synergists and one antagonist.
The first letter of the muscles has been provided.

1) This action happens at which joint?

_____

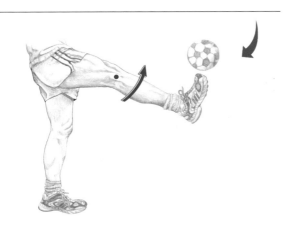

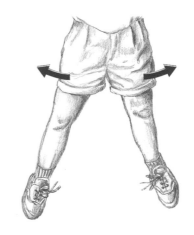

2) Action

_____

3) Synergists

V _____

V _____

4) Antagonist

G _____

5) Action

_____

6) Synergists

G _____

G _____

7) Antagonist

P _____

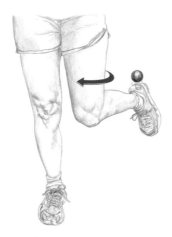

8) Action

_____

9) Synergists

G _____

P _____

10) Antagonist

B _____

Please list the action demonstrated, synergist(s) and antagonist(s).
The first letter of the muscles has been provided.

1) This action happens at which joint?

_____

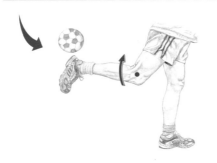

2) Action

_____

3) Synergists

B _____

G _____

4) Antagonist

R _____

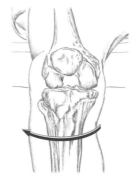

8) Action

_____

9) Synergist

B _____

10) Antagonists

S _____

S _____

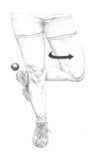

5) Action

_____

6) Synergists

P _____

I _____

7) Antagonist

A _____

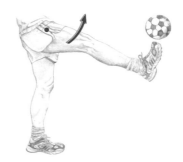

11) Action

_____

12) Synergists

T _____

S _____

13) Antagonist

G _____

154

Please identify the following muscles.

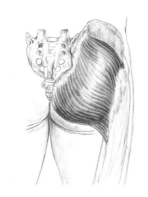

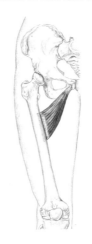

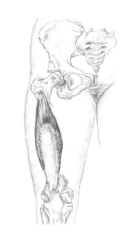

1) _____

2) _____

3) _____

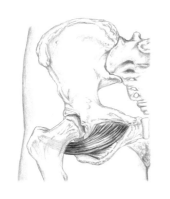

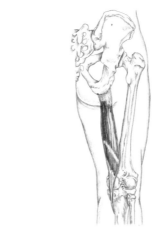

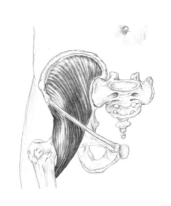

4) _____

5) _____

6) _____

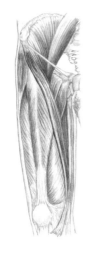

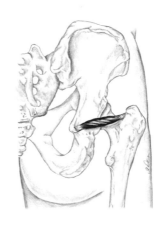

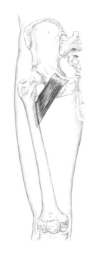

7) _____

8) _____

9) _____

What's the Muscle? #2

Please identify the following muscles.

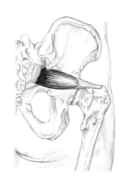

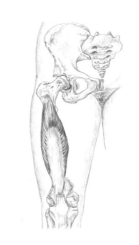

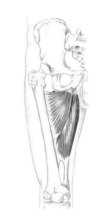

1) _____

2) _____

3) _____

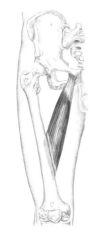

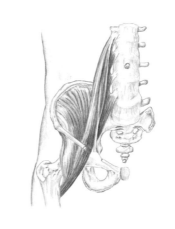

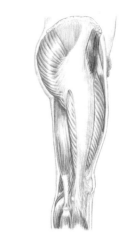

4) _____

5) _____

6) _____

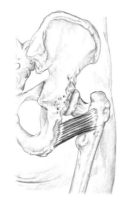

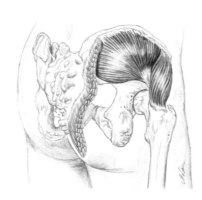

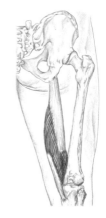

7) _____

8) _____

9) _____

156

Please identify the following muscles.

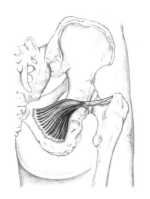

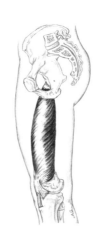

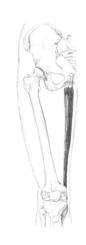

1) _____

2) _____

3) _____

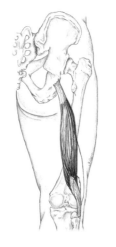

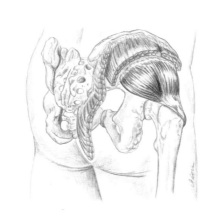

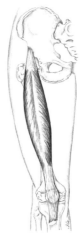

4) _____

5) _____

6) _____

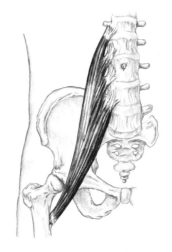

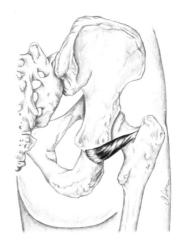

7) _____

8) _____

Please answer the following questions.

1) The muscles of the pelvis and thigh primarily create movement at the _____ and

    _____ joints.

2) _____ is the only quadriceps muscle that crosses two joints, the hip and knee.

3) Deep to the iliotibial tract, the _____ is the sole muscle of the lateral thigh.

4) To follow the path of the rectus femoris, it is helpful to draw an imaginary line from the

    _____ to the _____.

5) While your partner extends his knee, palpate just medial and proximal to the patella for the bulbous shape of the

    _____.

6) All three hamstrings share a common origin at the _____.

7) The hamstrings are located on the posterior thigh between the _____ and

    _____ muscles.

8) In which direction does biceps femoris rotate the hip? _____

9) The _____ is the more superficial of the medial hamstrings.

Let's Palpate!

Remember - there are no right or wrong answers here

Locate and explore the **hamstrings** on three individuals. Then write three words that describe what you feel.
(See p. 307-308 in *Trail Guide*)

Person #1 _____   Person #2 _____   Person #3 _____

_____   _____   _____

_____   _____   _____

_____   _____   _____

Matching

Match the origin and insertion to the correct muscle.

Origins
1) Anterior and lateral shaft of the femur

2) Anterior inferior iliac spine (AIIS)

3) Ischial tuberosity (2)

4) Ischial tuberosity, lateral lip of linea aspera

5) Lateral lip of linea aspera, gluteal tuberosity

6) Medial lip of linea aspera

Insertions
7) Head of the fibula

8) Posterior aspect of medial condyle of tibia

9) Proximal, medial shaft of the tibia at pes anserinus tendon

10) Tibial tuberosity (4)

Muscle	O	I
Biceps femoris	_____	_____
Rectus femoris	_____	_____
Semimembranosus	_____	_____
Semitendinosus	_____	_____
Vastus intermedius	_____	_____
Vastus lateralis	_____	_____
Vastus medialis	_____	_____

Shorten or Lengthen?

11) Passive flexion of the knee would _____ the vastus lateralis.

12) Passive tilting of the pelvis anteriorly would _____ the biceps femoris.

13) Passive medial rotation of the hip would _____ the semitendinosus.

14) Passive extension of the knee would _____ the vastus intermedius.

15) Passive lateral rotation of the flexed knee would _____ the biceps femoris.

16) Passive flexion of the hip would _____ the semimembranosus, but _____ the rectus femoris.

Please answer the following questions.

1) Of the three gluteal muscles, the _____ is the most posterior and superficial.

2) Which gluteal muscle has the ability to flex and extend the hip (but not simultaneously)?

    _____

3) Locating the coccyx, the posterior two inches of the iliac crest and gluteal tuberosity will help you to outline which muscle?

    _____

4) To palpate gluteus minimus, you will need to sink your fingers deep to which muscle? _____

5) To locate both gluteus medius and minimus in a sidelying position, you could ask your partner to perform which

    movement? _____

6) The adductor tendons form a connective tissue drape along the base of the pelvis extending from which two bony

    landmarks? _____

7) Located just anterior to the hamstrings, _____ is the most posterior of the adductor muscles.

8) Gracilis is the only adductor to cross which joint? _____

9) What are the two actions common to all the muscles of the adductor group?

    _____   _____

10) You will find the prominent tendon(s) of the gracilis and adductor longus extending off of, or nearby, which

    bony landmark? _____

11) Which muscle can be located just anterior to the prominent adductor tendon? _____

12) Which muscle can be located between the ischial tuberosity and the adductor tubercle?

    _____

Let's Palpate!

Remember - there are no right or wrong answers here

Locate and explore the **adductor group** on three individuals. Then write three words that describe what you feel.
(See p. 313-317 in *Trail Guide*)

Person #1 _____   Person #2 _____   Person #3 _____

_____   _____   _____

_____   _____   _____

_____   _____   _____

Matching

Match the origin and insertion to the correct muscle.

Origins

1) Coccyx, edge of sacrum, posterior iliac crest, sacrotuberous and sacroiliac ligaments

2) Gluteal surface of the ilium between anterior and inferior gluteal lines

3) Gluteal surface of the ilium between iliac crest and posterior and anterior gluteal lines

4) Inferior ramus of pubis

5) Inferior ramus of pubis and ramus of ischium

6) Inferior ramus of pubis, ramus of ischium and ischial tuberosity

7) Pubic tubercle

8) Superior ramus of pubis

Insertions

9) Anterior border of greater trochanter

10) Gluteal tuberosity and iliotibial tract

11) Greater trochanter

12) Medial lip of linea aspera

13) Medial lip of linea aspera and adductor tubercle

14) Pectineal line and medial lip of linea aspera

15) Pectineal line of femur

16) Proximal, medial shaft of tibia at pes anserinus tendon

Muscle	O	I
Adductor brevis	_____	_____
Adductor longus	_____	_____
Adductor magnus	_____	_____
Gluteus maximus	_____	_____
Gluteus medius	_____	_____
Gluteus minimus	_____	_____
Gracilis	_____	_____
Pectineus	_____	_____

Shorten or Lengthen?

17) Passive abduction of the hip would _____ the adductor brevis and longus.

18) Passive lateral rotation of the hip would _____ the gluteus maximus.

19) Passive extension of the hip would _____ the posterior fibers of the adductor magnus.

20) Passive adduction of the hip would _____ the gluteus medius.

21) Passive lateral rotation of the hip would _____ the gluteus minimus.

22) Passive extension and lateral rotation of the hip would _____ the gracilis.

23) Passive medial rotation of the hip would _____ the adductors.

24) Passive flexion of the hip would _____ the gluteus maximus.

Please answer the following questions.

1) Which muscle is most accessible between the upper fibers of the rectus femoris and gluteus medius?

   _____

2) Which cablelike band of fascia can be isolated just anterior to the biceps femoris tendon?

   _____

3) In order to feel the tensor fasciae latae contract, position your partner in a supine position and ask him to perform

   what action? _____

4) Which muscle stretches from the anterior superior iliac spine (ASIS) to the medial knee?

   _____

5) The proximal fibers of the sartorius are just lateral to which artery? _____

6) Which three tendons blend together to become the pes anserinus tendon?

   _____ _____ _____

7) Which muscle lies superficial to the sciatic nerve and can compress the nerve if overcontracted?

   _____

8) To locate the piriformis, form a "T" with which three bony landmarks?

   _____ _____ _____

9) Which rectangular muscle can be isolated by placing your fingerpads between the distal, posterior aspect of the

   greater trochanter and the ischial tuberosity? _____

10) Which muscle spans from the anterior surface of the lumbar vertebrae to the lesser trochanter?

   _____

11) To access the psoas major, place your fingerpads between the _____ and _____
    before slowly compressing toward the muscle.

12) What are some ways to ensure your partner's comfort during palpation of the psoas major?

   _____ _____

   _____ _____

   _____ _____

13) What action could you ask your partner to perform to confirm that you have located the psoas major?

   _____

Pelvis and Thigh, Muscle Group #3
TFL, Sartorius, Lateral Rotators and Iliopsoas

Matching

Match the origin and insertion to the correct muscle.

Origins

1) Anterior superior iliac spine (ASIS)

2) Anterior surface of sacrum

3) Body and transverse process of first lumbar vertebra

4) Bodies and transverse processes of lumbar vertebrae

5) Iliac crest, posterior to the ASIS

6) Iliac fossa

7) Ischial spine

8) Ischial tuberosity

9) Lateral border of ischial tuberosity

10) Obturator membrane and inferior surface of obturator foramen

11) Superior and inferior rami of pubis

Insertions

12) Greater trochanter

13) Iliotibial tract

14) Lesser trochanter (2)

15) Medial surface of greater trochanter

16) Intertrochanteric crest, between the greater and lesser trochanters

17) Proximal, medial shaft of tibia at pes anserinus tendon

18) Superior ramus of pubis

19) Trochanteric fossa of femur

20) Upper border of greater trochanter (2)

Muscle	O	I
Gemellus inferior	_____	_____
Gemellus superior	_____	_____
Iliacus	_____	_____
Obturator externus	_____	_____
Obturator internus	_____	_____
Piriformis	_____	_____
Psoas major	_____	_____
Psoas minor	_____	_____
Quadratus femoris	_____	_____
Sartorius	_____	_____
Tensor fasciae latae	_____	_____

Let's Palpate!

Remember - there are no right or wrong answers here

Locate and explore the **tensor fasciae latae and iliotibial tract** on three individuals. Then write three words that describe what you feel. (See p. 318-319 in *Trail Guide*)

Person #1 _____

Person #2 _____

Person #3 _____

_____   _____   _____

_____   _____   _____

_____   _____   _____

Shorten or Lengthen?

1) Passive medial rotation of the flexed knee would _____ the sartorius.

2) Passive adduction of the hip would _____ the tensor fasciae latae.

3) Passive extension of the hip would _____ the iliopsoas muscles.

4) Passive lateral rotation of the hip would _____ the piriformis.

5) Passive extension of the hip would _____ the psoas major.

6) Passive flexion of the hip would _____ the sartorius.

7) Passive lateral rotation of the hip would _____ the iliacus.

8) Passive medial rotation of the hip would _____ the tensor fasciae latae.

9) Passive medial rotation of the hip would _____ the quadratus femoris.

10) Passive abduction of the hip would _____ the sartorius.

Let's Palpate!   *Remember - there are no right or wrong answers here*

Locate and explore the **psoas major** on three individuals. Then write three words that describe what you feel.
(See p. 326-328 in *Trail Guide*)

Person #1 _____   Person #2 _____   Person #3 _____

_____   _____   _____

_____   _____   _____

_____   _____   _____

Please identify the following structures.

CHOICES
Adductor longus (2)
Femoral artery
Femoral nerve
Femoral vein
Great saphenous vein
Inguinal ligament (2)
Inguinal lymph nodes
Sartorius (2)

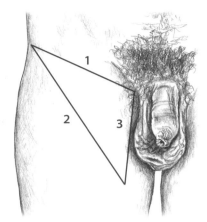

1) _____

2) _____

3) _____

The three borders of the femoral triangle

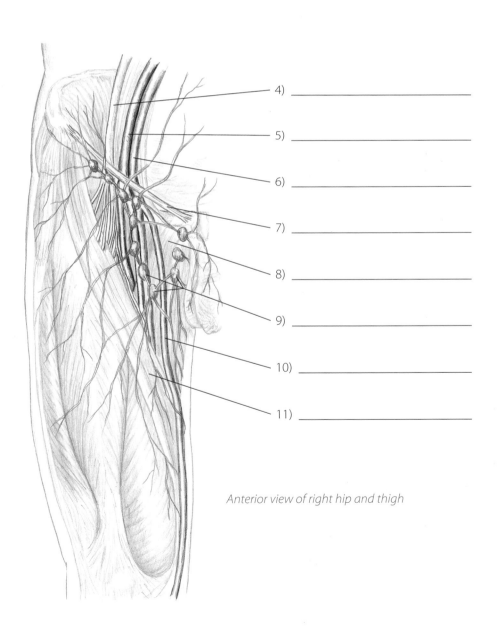

4) _____

5) _____

6) _____

7) _____

8) _____

9) _____

10) _____

11) _____

Anterior view of right hip and thigh

1) _____

2) _____

3) _____

Please identify the following structures.

Color Them!

CHOICES

Anterior longitudinal ligament
Anterior sacroiliac ligament
Hamstrings tendon
Iliolumbar ligament (2)
Inguinal ligament
Posterior sacrococcygeal ligaments
Posterior sacroiliac ligaments
Pubic symphysis
Sacrospinous ligament (2)
Sacrotuberous ligament (2)
Supraspinous ligament

4) _____

5) _____

6) _____

7) _____

Anterior view of right side of pelvis

8) _____

9) _____

Posterior view of pelvis

10) _____

11) _____

12) _____

14) _____   13) _____

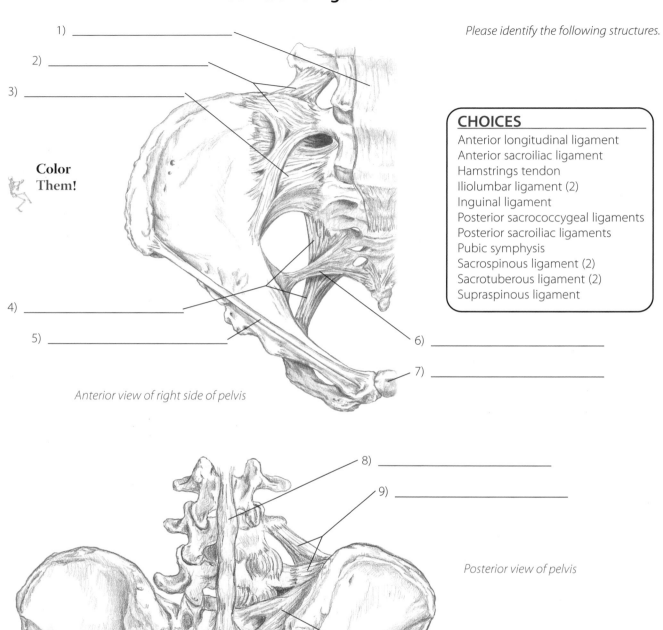

Please identify the following structures.

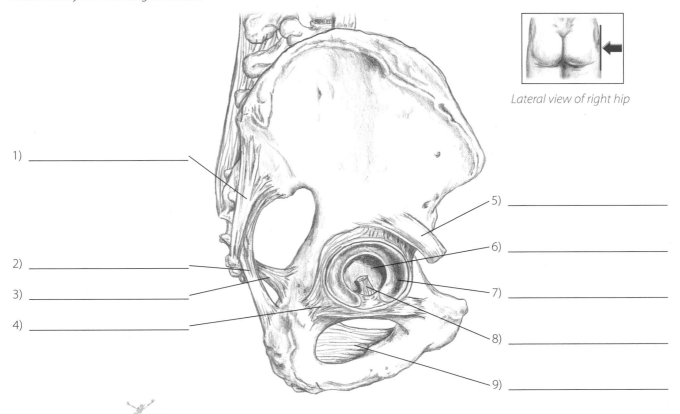

Lateral view of right hip

1) _____

2) _____

3) _____

4) _____

5) _____

6) _____

7) _____

8) _____

9) _____

Color Them!

CHOICES

Acetabulum
Anterior sacroiliac ligament
Articular capsule of coxal joint
Lunate surface of acetabulum
Obturator membrane (2)
Posterior sacroiliac ligaments
Pubic symphysis
Round ligament
    (ligamentum capitis femoris - cut)
Sacrospinous ligament (2)
Sacrotuberous ligament (2)
Tendon of rectus femoris (cut)

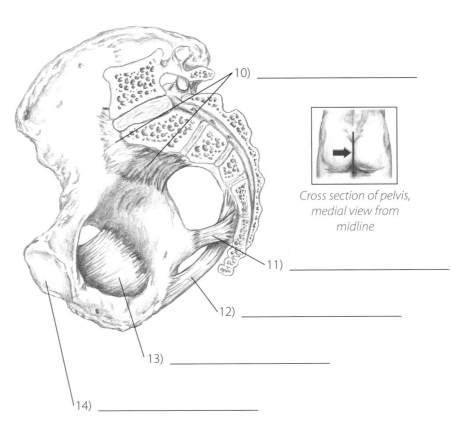

Cross section of pelvis, medial view from midline

10) _____

11) _____

12) _____

13) _____

14) _____

Please identify the following structures.

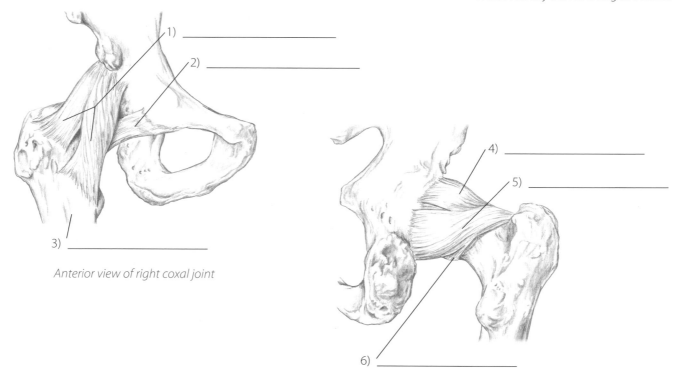

1) _____

2) _____

3) _____

Anterior view of right coxal joint

4) _____

5) _____

6) _____

Posterior view of right coxal joint

**Color
Them!**

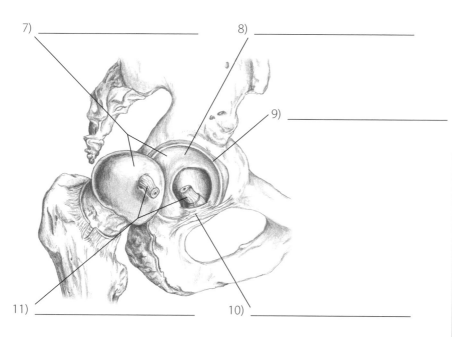

7) _____

8) _____

9) _____

11) _____

10) _____

Lateral view of right coxal joint, femur reflected

CHOICES

Acetabular labrum
Articular cartilage
Femur
Iliofemoral ligament (2)
Ischiofemoral ligament
Lunate surface of acetabulum
Pubofemoral ligament
Round ligament
    (ligamentum capitis femoris - cut)
Transverse acetabular ligament
Zona orbicularis

Please answer the following questions.

1) The inguinal ligament stretches from the _____ to the _____.

2) Which three vessels pass through the femoral triangle?

   _____   _____

   _____

3) Where should you position your fingers to feel the pulse of the femoral artery?

   _____

4) What structure spans from the ischial tuberosity to the edge of the sacrum? _____

5) The _____ ligaments help to reinforce the union of the sacrum and the ilium.

6) The transverse processes of the fourth and fifth lumbar vertebrae and the posterior iliac crest are helpful landmarks in

   finding which ligament? _____

7) Which structure spans from the lower lumbar vertebrae, between the ischial tuberosity and greater

   trochanter and down the posterior thigh? _____

8) Which structure reduces friction between the greater trochanter and the gluteus maximus?

   _____

Let's Palpate! _____

Remember - there are no right or wrong answers here

Locate and explore the **sacrotuberous ligament** on three individuals. Then write three words that describe
what you feel. (See p. 334 in *Trail Guide*)

Person #1 _____   Person #2 _____   Person #3 _____

_____   _____   _____

_____   _____   _____

_____   _____   _____

Notes

p. 338

Please identify the following structures.

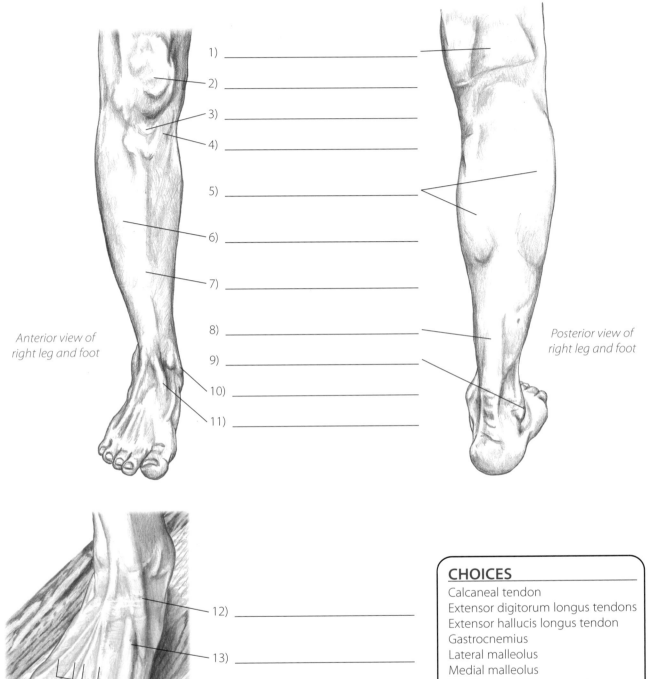

1) _____

2) _____

3) _____

4) _____

5) _____

6) _____

7) _____

8) _____

9) _____

10) _____

11) _____

12) _____

13) _____

14) _____

*Anterior view of
right leg and foot*

*Posterior view of
right leg and foot*

Dorsal view of right foot

CHOICES

Calcaneal tendon
Extensor digitorum longus tendons
Extensor hallucis longus tendon
Gastrocnemius
Lateral malleolus
Medial malleolus
Patella
Pes anserinus attachment site
Popliteal fossa
Shaft of the tibia
Tibial tuberosity
Tibialis anterior
Tibialis anterior tendon (2)

Please answer the following questions.

1) The anatomical name for the knee is the _____ joint.

2) Medial and lateral rotation of the knee can occur when the knee is in a _____ position.

3) The bone running superficially down the anterior surface of the leg is the _____ while

   the bone buried deep to the surrounding muscle tissue on the leg is the _____.

4) The patella seems to disappear when the knee is flexed. It sinks between which two landmarks?

   _____   _____

5) The bony landmark located distal to the patella is the _____.

6) The connective tissue structure connecting the patella to the tibial tuberosity is the _____.

7) The head of the fibula is the attachment site for which two muscles and ligament?

   _____   _____   _____

8) Which portion of the tibial plateaus can be accessed? _____

9) Which three tendons form the pes anserinus tendon?

   _____   _____   _____

10) With the knee fully extended and the patella shifted medially or laterally, what structures can be found deep

   to the patella? _____

11) To locate the lateral epicondyle of the femur you would need to palpate deep to what structure?

   _____

12) Which landmark is located proximal to the medial epicondyle of the femur, and the tendon of what muscle attaches to it?

   _____   _____

Please identify the following bones. (Questions 1-8)

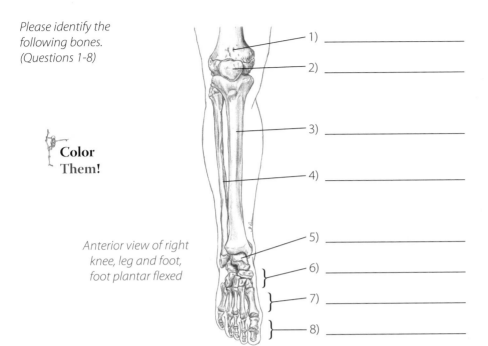

Color Them!

Anterior view of right knee, leg and foot, foot plantar flexed

1) _____
2) _____
3) _____
4) _____
5) _____
6) _____
7) _____
8) _____

CHOICES

Femur
Fibula
Fossa of lateral malleolus
Head of the fibula
Lateral condyle (2)
Lateral malleolus (2)
Medial and lateral
    intercondylar tubercles
Medial condyle
Medial malleolus (2)
Metatarsals
Patella
Phalanges
Soleal line
Talus
Tarsals
Tibia
Tibial tuberosity

Please identify the following bony landmarks. (Questions 9-20)

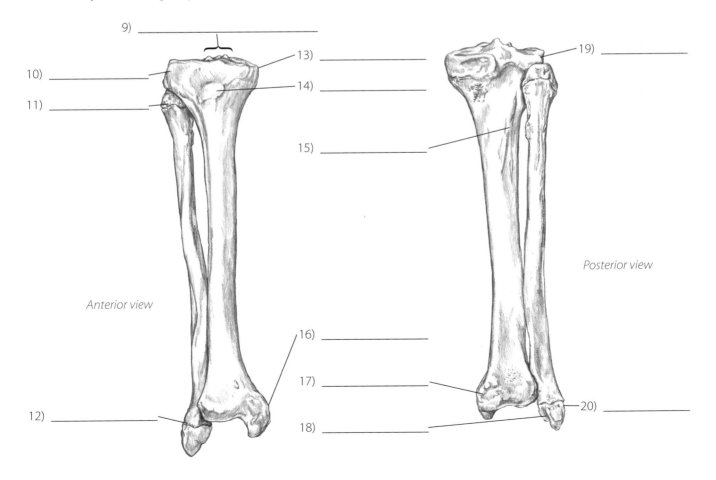

9) _____
10) _____
11) _____
13) _____
14) _____
15) _____
16) _____
17) _____
18) _____
19) _____
20) _____
12) _____

Anterior view

Posterior view

Please identify the following structures.

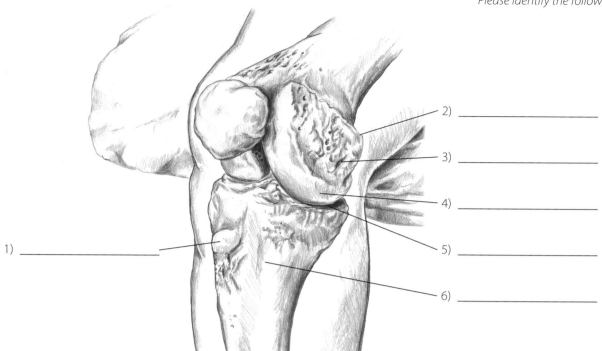

2) _____

3) _____

4) _____

1) _____

5) _____

6) _____

Anterior/medial view of right knee

CHOICES

Adductor tubercle
Head of the fibula
Lateral condyle
Lateral epicondyle
Medial condyle
Medial epicondyle
Pes anserinus attachment site
Shaft of the tibia
Tibial plateau (2)
Tibial tubercle
Tibial tuberosity (2)

Color Them!

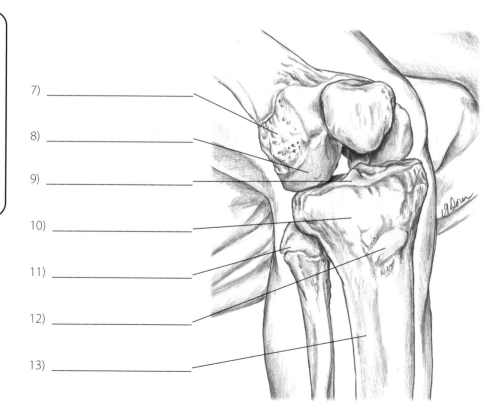

7) _____

8) _____

9) _____

10) _____

11) _____

12) _____

13) _____

Anterior/lateral view of right knee

Please identify the following structures.

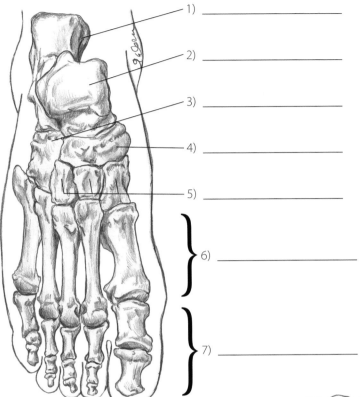

1) _____

2) _____

3) _____

4) _____

5) _____

6) _____

7) _____

Dorsal view of right foot

CHOICES

Calcaneus (2)
Cuboid (2)
Lateral, middle and
    medial cuneiforms (2)
Metatarsals (2)
Navicular (2)
Phalanges (2)
Sesamoid bones
Talus (2)

**Color
Them!**

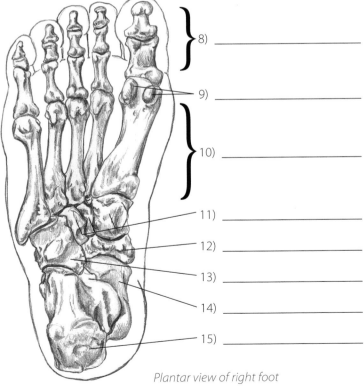

8) _____

9) _____

10) _____

11) _____

12) _____

13) _____

14) _____

15) _____

Plantar view of right foot

*Please identify the following structures. Numbers in **bold** indicate bones.*

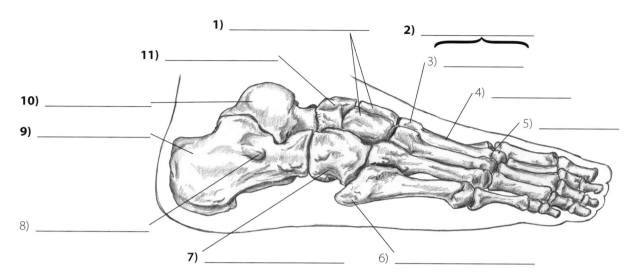

1) _____

2) _____

11) _____

3) _____

10) _____

4) _____

9) _____

5) _____

8) _____

7) _____

6) _____

Lateral view of right foot

CHOICES

Base (2)
Base of first metatarsal
Calcaneus (2)
Cuboid
Head (2)
Head of the talus
Lateral and middle cuneiform
Medial cuneiform
Medial tubercle of talus
Metatarsals

Navicular
Navicular tubercle
Peroneal trochlea
Phalanges
Shaft (2)
Sustentaculum tali
Talus (2)
Trochlea of the talus
Tuberosity of calcaneus
Tuberosity of fifth metatarsal

Color Them!

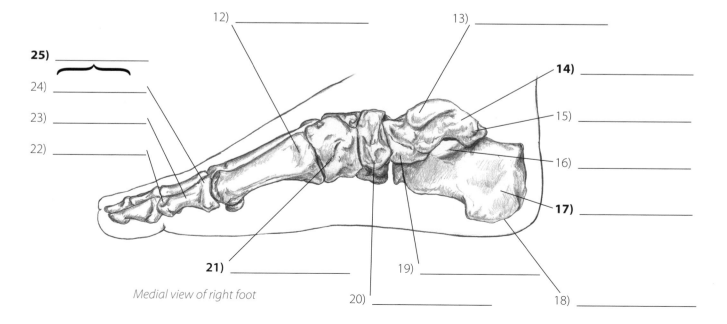

12) _____

13) _____

25) _____

14) _____

24) _____

15) _____

23) _____

16) _____

22) _____

17) _____

21) _____

19) _____

20) _____

18) _____

Medial view of right foot

Please identify the following structures.

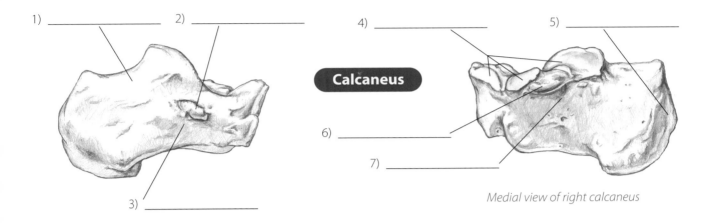

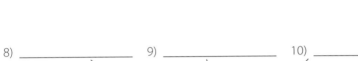

Calcaneus

1) _____

2) _____

3) _____

Lateral view of right calcaneus

4) _____

5) _____

6) _____

7) _____

Medial view of right calcaneus

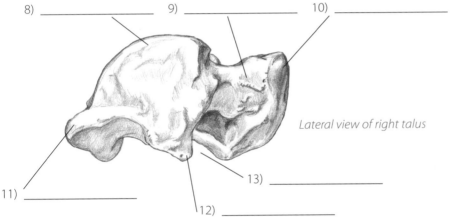

8) _____

9) _____

10) _____

11) _____

12) _____

13) _____

Lateral view of right talus

CHOICES

Articular surfaces for talus
Body
Groove for flexor hallucis
 longus tendon
Groove for peroneus
 longus tendon
Head (2)
Lateral process
Lateral tubercle
Medial tubercle
Neck (2)
Peroneal trochlea
Sustentaculum tali
Tarsal sinus
Trochlea (2)
Tuberosity

Talus

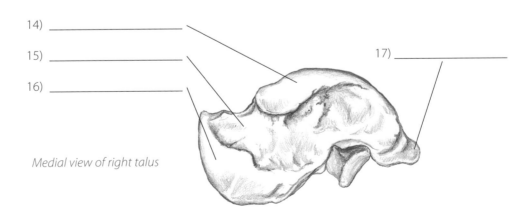

14) _____

15) _____

16) _____

17) _____

Medial view of right talus

Please answer the following questions.

1) The bone at the heel of the foot is the _____, while the bone that articulates with the

   tibia and fibula is the _____.

2) The tarsals are most accessible along which surface of the foot? _____

3) As you palpate both malleoli of the ankle, which extends further distally? _____

4) How would you passively position the foot to shorten the surrounding tissue of the medial malleolar groove?

   _____

5) In which direction from the medial malleolus would you move your thumb to locate the sustentaculum tali? And
   approximately how far would you move?

   _____   _____

6) The head of the talus can be located between which two bony landmarks?

   _____   _____

7) How would you passively position the foot to best locate the trochlea of the talus?

   _____

8) The proximal end of the first metatarsal articulates with which bone? _____

9) Which two superficial surfaces of the first metatarsal are easily accessible?

   _____   _____

10) Spelled out, what do the acronyms "pip" and "dip" stand for?

    _____   _____

11) The tuberosity of the fifth metatarsal is the attachment site for which muscle? _____

12) Which tendon could you follow along the dorsal surface of the ankle to locate the medial cuneiform?

    _____

13) Locate the navicular and tuberosity of the fifth metatarsal. Which is situated further distally on the foot?

    _____

14) Between which two bony landmarks can you draw a line to locate the cuboid?

    _____   _____

Please identify the following structures.

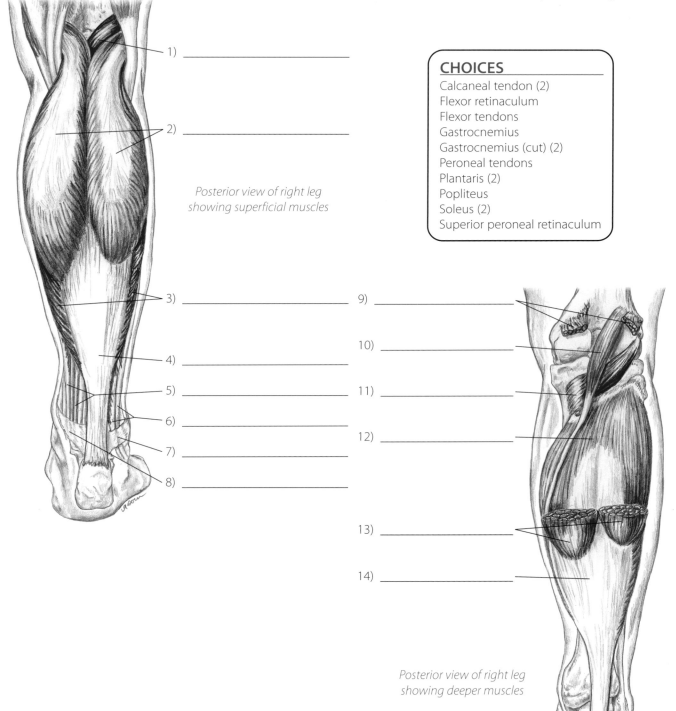

1) _____

2) _____

*Posterior view of right leg
showing superficial muscles*

CHOICES

Calcaneal tendon (2)
Flexor retinaculum
Flexor tendons
Gastrocnemius
Gastrocnemius (cut) (2)
Peroneal tendons
Plantaris (2)
Popliteus
Soleus (2)
Superior peroneal retinaculum

3) _____

4) _____

5) _____

6) _____

7) _____

8) _____

9) _____

10) _____

11) _____

12) _____

13) _____

14) _____

*Posterior view of right leg
showing deeper muscles*

Please identify the following structures.

1) _____

2) _____

3) _____

4) _____

5) _____

6) _____

CHOICES

Extensor digitorum longus (2)
Extensor hallucis longus
Gastrocnemius (2)
Peroneus brevis (2)
Peroneus longus (2)
Soleus (2)
Tibialis anterior (2)

*Lateral view of
right leg and foot*

7) _____

8) _____

9) _____

10) _____

11) _____

12) _____

13) _____

*Anterior view of
right leg and foot*

Please identify the following structures.

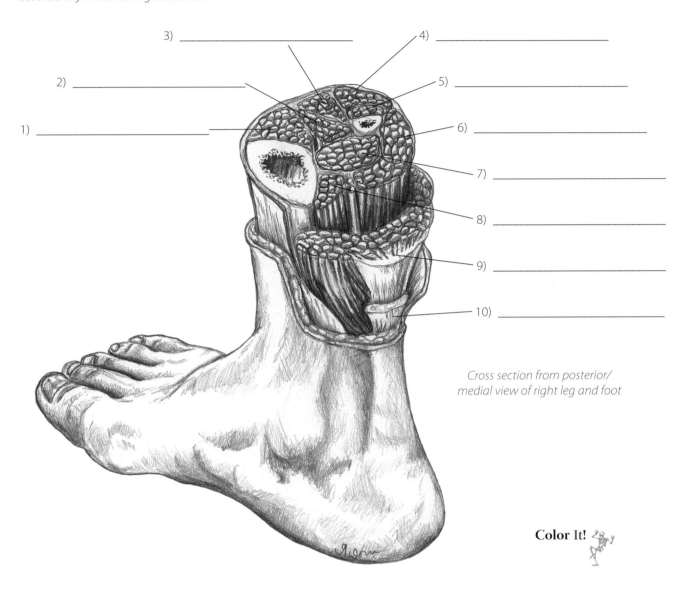

3) _____

4) _____

2) _____

5) _____

1) _____

6) _____

7) _____

8) _____

9) _____

10) _____

Cross section from posterior/ medial view of right leg and foot

Color It!

CHOICES

Calcaneal tendon
Extensor digitorum longus
Extensor hallucis longus
Flexor digitorum longus
Flexor hallucis longus
Peroneus brevis
Peroneus longus
Soleus
Tibialis anterior
Tibialis posterior

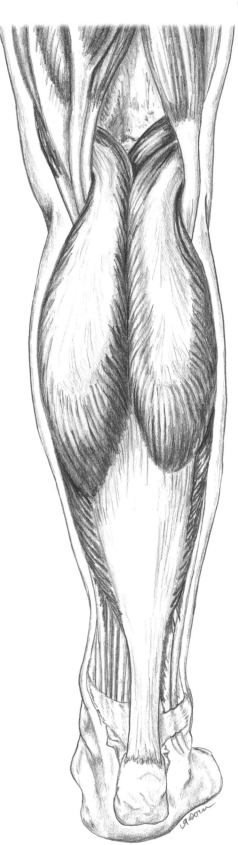

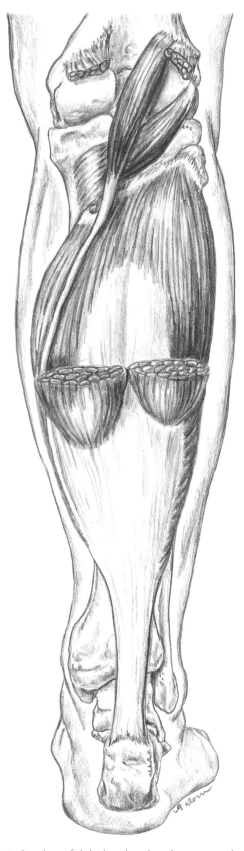

Using different colors, please fill in and label the muscles and other structures listed below.

Calcaneal tendon
Flexor tendons
Gastrocnemius
Gastrocnemius (cut)
Peroneal tendons
Plantaris
Popliteus
Soleus

Posterior view of right leg showing superficial muscles

Posterior view of right leg showing deeper muscles

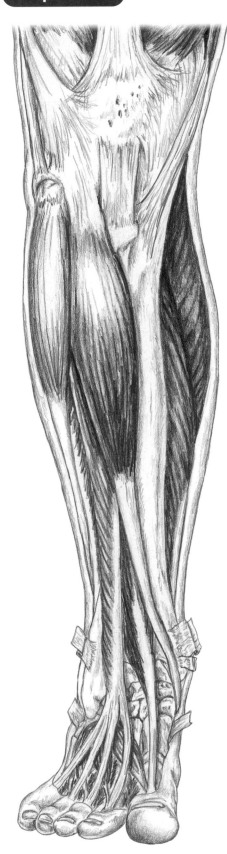

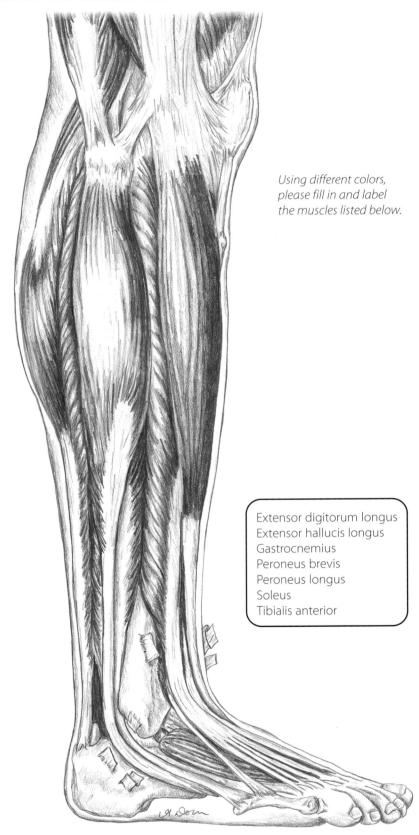

Using different colors, please fill in and label the muscles listed below.

Extensor digitorum longus
Extensor hallucis longus
Gastrocnemius
Peroneus brevis
Peroneus longus
Soleus
Tibialis anterior

Anterior view of right leg and foot

Lateral view of right leg and foot

Please list the action demonstrated, two synergists and one antagonist.
The first letter of the muscles has been provided.

1) This action happens at which joint?

_____

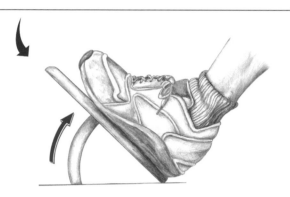

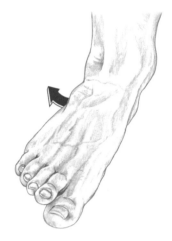

2) Action

_____

3) Synergists

T _____

E _____

4) Antagonist

F _____

5) Action

_____

6) Synergists

P _____

P _____

7) Antagonist

T _____

8) Action

_____

9) Synergists

F _____

F _____

10) Antagonist

L _____

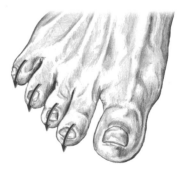

Please list the action demonstrated, two synergists and one antagonist.
The first letter of the muscles has been provided.

1) This action happens at which three joints?

_____

_____

_____

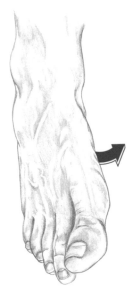

5) Action

_____

6) Synergists

T _____

F _____

7) Antagonist

E _____

2) Action

_____

3) Synergists

E _____

L _____

4) Antagonist

F _____

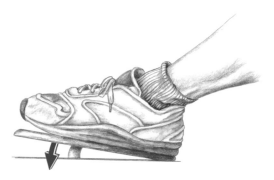

8) Action

_____

9) Synergists

S _____

T _____

10) Antagonist

E _____

Please identify the following muscles.

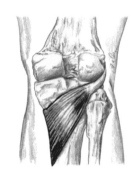

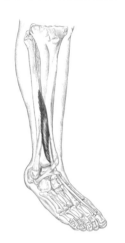

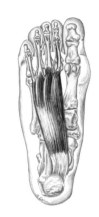

1) _____

2) _____

3) _____

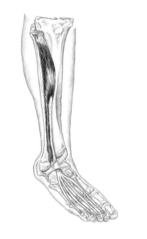

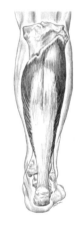

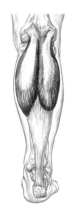

4) _____

5) _____

6) _____

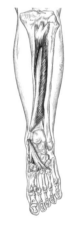

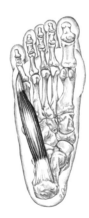

7) _____

8) _____

186

Please identify the following muscles.

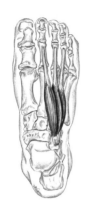

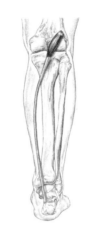

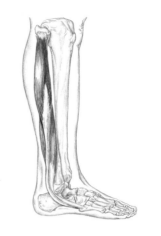

1) _____

2) _____

3) _____

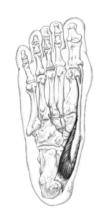

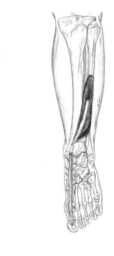

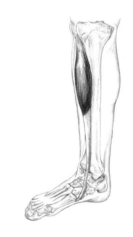

4) _____

5) _____

6) _____

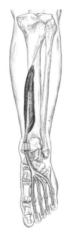

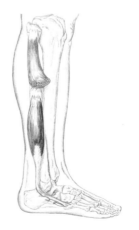

7) _____

8) _____

Please answer the following questions.

1) What are the two muscles that form the "triceps surae?" _____ _____

2) The gastrocnemius extends halfway down the leg before blending into which band of connective tissue?

   _____

3) What common action could you ask your partner to do to contract his gastrocnemius and soleus?

   _____

4) Palpate both bellies of the gastrocnemius. Which head extends further distally?

   _____

5) Although the gastrocnemius and soleus are located on the posterior leg, you can palpate them on the leg's anterior

   surface by sliding _____ off the _____.

6) The muscle belly accessed between the gastrocnemius heads, in the popliteal space, is the _____.

7) The belly of the plantaris can be distinguished by its _____-wide belly that runs at an

   _____ angle.

8) Which muscle is the deepest of the popliteal space? _____

9) When the knee is extended, the popliteus plays what important role?

   _____

10) To access the popliteus' tendinous attachment you need to push the overlying edge of which muscles to the side?

    _____ _____

11) The peroneal muscles are located on the _____ side of the leg and lie between which

    two muscles? _____ _____

12) What are two bony landmarks that can help you isolate the peroneal bellies?

    _____ _____

13) What action could you ask your partner to perform to feel the peroneals tighten?

    _____

Matching

Match the origin and insertion to the correct muscle.

Origins

1) Distal two-thirds of lateral fibula

2) Lateral epicondyle of the femur

3) Lateral condyle of the femur

4) Condyles of the femur, posterior surfaces

5) Proximal two-thirds of lateral fibula

6) Soleal line, posterior surface of tibia
and proximal, posterior surface of fibula

Muscle	O	I
Gastrocnemius	_____	_____
Peroneus brevis	_____	_____
Peroneus longus	_____	_____
Plantaris	_____	_____
Popliteus	_____	_____
Soleus	_____	_____

Insertions

7) Base of the first metatarsal and medial cuneiform

8) Calcaneus via calcaneal tendon (3)

9) Proximal, posterior aspect of tibia

10) Tuberosity of fifth metatarsal

Shorten or Lengthen?

11) Passive dorsiflexion of the ankle would _____ the soleus.

12) Passive lateral rotation of the knee would _____ the popliteus.

13) Passive inversion of the foot would _____ the peroneus longus.

14) Passive flexion of the knee would _____ the gastrocnemius.

Let's Palpate!   *Remember - there are no right or wrong answers here*

Locate and explore the **gastrocnemius and soleus** on three individuals. Then write three words that describe what you feel. (See p. 364-366 in *Trail Guide*)

Person #1 _____

Person #2 _____

Person #3 _____

_____

_____

_____

_____

_____

_____

_____

_____

_____

Please answer the following questions.

1) The tibialis anterior belly can be easily located lateral to which bony landmark? _____

2) To feel the tibialis anterior belly contract, you could ask your partner to perform which action?

   _____

3) Along the ankle's dorsal surface, the extensor hallucis longus and extensor digitorum longus both pass underneath

   which band of connective tissue? _____

4) The flexors of the ankle and toes are virtually inaccessible, except on the medial side of the leg between which
   two structures?

   _____   _____

5) Please complete the following for the mnemonic device "**T**om, **D**ick **AN**' **H**arry".

   T_____   _____

   _____   **D**_____   _____

   _____   **A**_____

   _____   **N**_____

   _____   **H**_____   _____

6) What action at the toes could you ask your partner to perform to feel contraction of all the flexor bellies?

   _____

7) The dorsal surface of the foot is home to which muscle that extends down to the second, third and fourth toes?

   _____

8) The first layer of muscles on the foot's plantar surface is deep to which connective tissue structure?

   _____

9) Which tendons do you need to palpate beneath to locate the belly of the extensor digitorum brevis?

   _____

10) What two structures are helpful in isolating the flexor digitorum brevis?

   _____   _____

11) Not everyone has the coordination to abduct their first toe. What is another action your partner could do to

   contract the abductor hallucis? _____

12) Which three points of contact form a triangle with the three arches of the foot?

   _____   _____   _____

Matching

Match the origin and insertion to the correct muscle.

Origins

1) Proximal anterior shaft of fibula and interosseous membrane

2) Proximal lateral surface of tibia and interosseous membrane

3) Middle anterior surface of fibula and interosseous membrane

4) Middle half of posterior fibula

5) Middle posterior surface of tibia

6) Proximal posterior shaft of tibia, proximal fibula and interosseous membrane

Muscle	O	I
Extensor digitorum longus	_____	_____
Extensor hallucis longus	_____	_____
Flexor digitorum longus	_____	_____
Flexor hallucis longus	_____	_____
Tibialis anterior	_____	_____
Tibialis posterior	_____	_____

Insertions

7) Distal phalange of first toe (2)

8) Distal phalanges of second through fifth toes

9) Medial cuneiform and base of the first metatarsal

10) Middle and distal phalanges of second through fifth toes

11) Navicular, cuneiforms, cuboid and bases of second through fourth metatarsals

Shorten or Lengthen?

12) Passive flexion of the fifth toe would _____ the abductor digiti minimi.

13) Passive eversion of the foot would _____ the tibialis posterior.

14) Passive dorsiflexion of the ankle would _____ the extensor digitorum longus.

15) Passive eversion of the foot would _____ the tibialis anterior.

Let's Palpate!

Remember - there are no right or wrong answers here

Locate and explore the **tibialis anterior** on three individuals. Then write three words that describe what you feel. (See p. 371-372 in *Trail Guide*)

Person #1 _____   Person #2 _____   Person #3 _____

_____   _____   _____

_____   _____   _____

_____   _____   _____

Please identify the following structures.

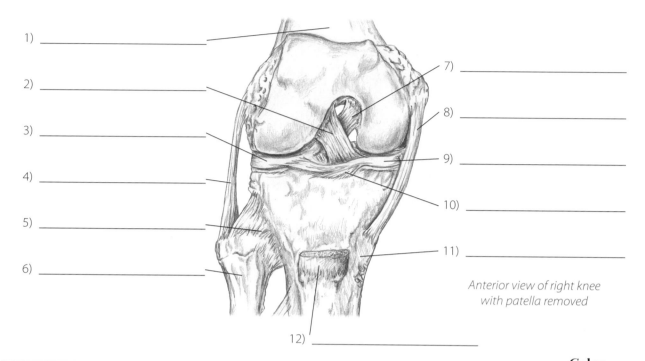

1) _____

2) _____

3) _____

4) _____

5) _____

6) _____

7) _____

8) _____

9) _____

10) _____

11) _____

12) _____

*Anterior view of right knee
with patella removed*

CHOICES

Anterior cruciate ligament (2)
Anterior ligament
    of head of the fibula
Femur
Fibula
Fibular collateral
    ligament (2)
Lateral meniscus (2)
Medial meniscus (2)
Patellar ligament (cut)
Popliteus tendon (cut)
Posterior cruciate
    ligament (2)
Posterior ligament
    of head of the fibula
Posterior meniscofemoral
    ligament
Tibia
Tibial collateral
    ligament (2)
Transverse ligament of knee

**Color
Them!**

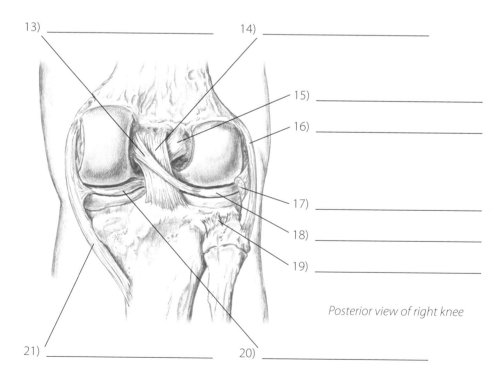

13) _____

14) _____

15) _____

16) _____

17) _____

18) _____

19) _____

20) _____

21) _____

Posterior view of right knee

192

Please identify the following structures.

CHOICES

Anterior cruciate ligament (cut)
Anterior ligament of head of the fibula
Anterior talofibular ligament (cut)
Anterior tibiofibular ligament
Biceps femoris tendon (cut)
Cruciate ligaments (cut)
Fibula
Fibular collateral ligament (cut)
Iliotibial tract (cut)
Interosseous membrane
Lateral meniscus
Medial meniscus
Patellar ligament (cut)
Posterior cruciate ligament (cut)
Posterior meniscofemoral ligament (cut)
Tibia
Tibial collateral ligament (cut)

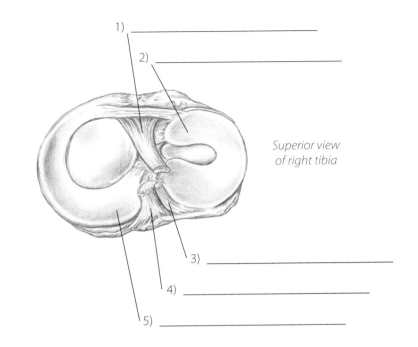

1) _____

2) _____

Superior view of right tibia

3) _____

4) _____

5) _____

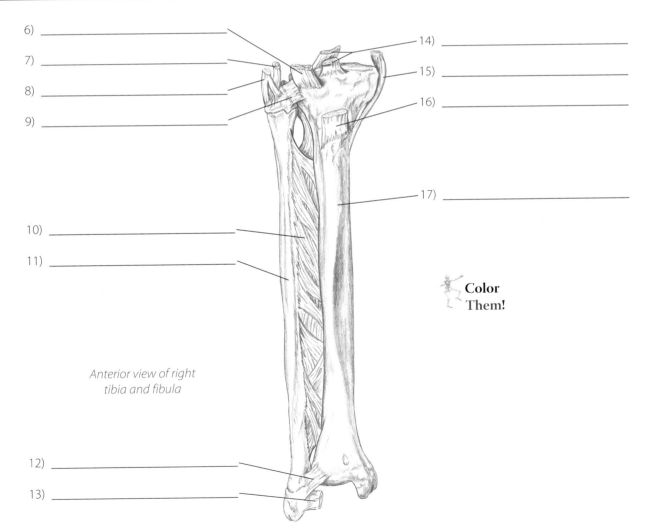

6) _____

7) _____

8) _____

9) _____

14) _____

15) _____

16) _____

17) _____

10) _____

11) _____

Color Them!

Anterior view of right tibia and fibula

12) _____

13) _____

Please identify the following structures.

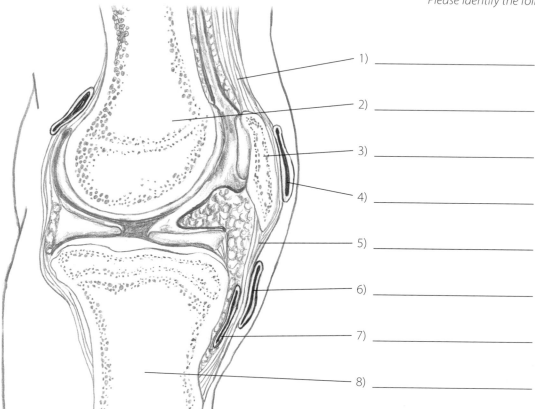

1) _____

2) _____

3) _____

4) _____

5) _____

6) _____

7) _____

8) _____

Lateral cross section of knee

CHOICES

Common peroneal nerve
Deep infrapatellar bursa
Femur
Gastrocnemius
Hamstrings
Lesser saphenous vein
Patella
Patellar ligament
Popliteal artery and vein
Prepatellar bursa
Quadriceps femoris tendon
Subcutaneous
    infrapatellar bursa
Tibia
Tibial nerve

9) _____

10) _____

11) _____

12) _____

13) _____

14) _____

🏃 **Color It!**

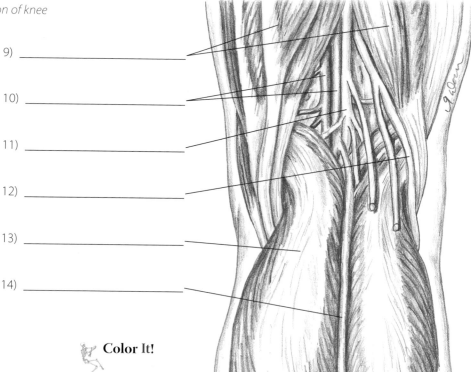

Posterior view of right knee

194

Please identify the following structures.

1) _____

2) _____

3) _____

4) _____

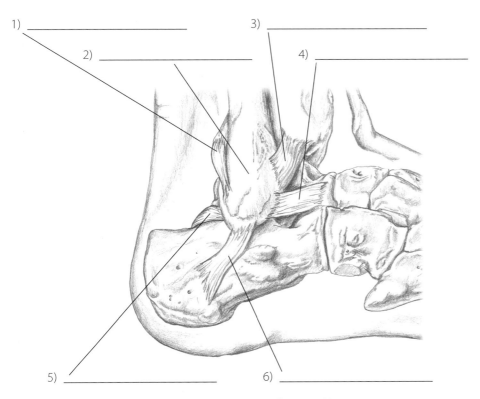

5) _____

6) _____

Lateral view of right ankle

CHOICES

Anterior talofibular ligament
Anterior tibiofibular ligament
Anterior tibiotalar ligament
Calcaneofibular ligament
Deltoid ligament
Lateral malleolus
Medial malleolus
Navicular
Posterior talofibular ligament
Posterior tibiofibular ligament
Posterior tibiotalar ligament
Sustentaculum tali
Tibiocalcaneal ligament
Tibionavicular ligament

**Color
Them!**

7) _____ :

8) _____

9) _____

10) _____

11) _____

12) _____

13) _____

14) _____

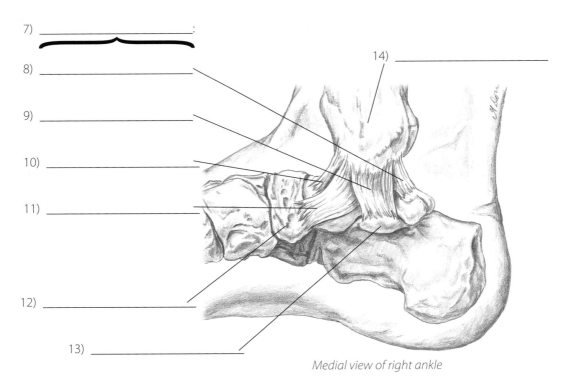

Medial view of right ankle

Please identify the following structures.

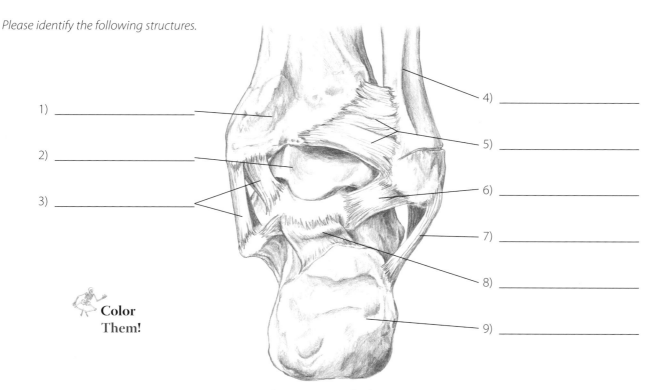

1) _____

2) _____

3) _____

4) _____

5) _____

6) _____

7) _____

8) _____

9) _____

Color
Them!

Posterior view of right ankle

CHOICES

Calcaneofibular ligament
Calcaneus
Deltoid ligament
Fibula
Interosseous talocalcaneal
   ligament
Lateral talocalcaneal ligament
Navicular
Posterior talocalcaneal ligament (2)
Posterior talofibular ligament
Posterior tibiofibular ligament
Talonavicular ligament
Talus (2)
Tibia

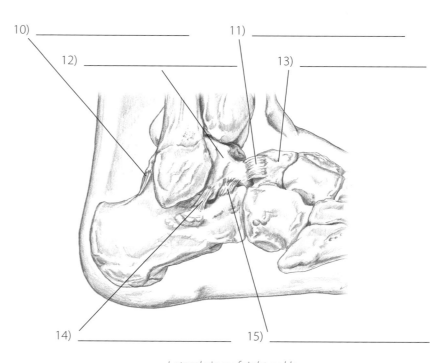

10) _____

11) _____

12) _____

13) _____

14) _____

15) _____

Lateral view of right ankle

Please identify the following structures.

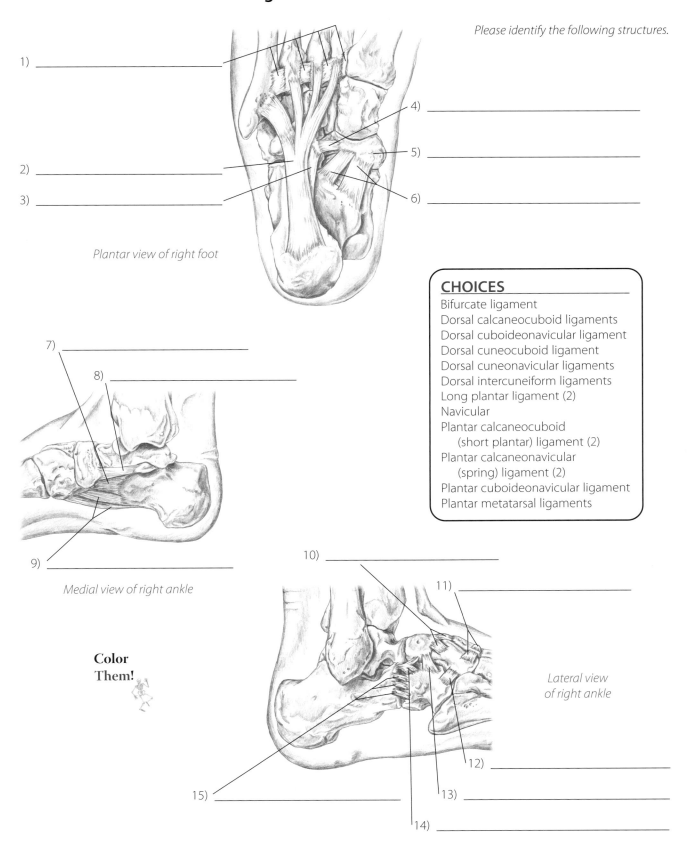

1) _____

2) _____

3) _____

Plantar view of right foot

4) _____

5) _____

6) _____

7) _____

8) _____

9) _____

Medial view of right ankle

Color Them!

10) _____

11) _____

Lateral view of right ankle

12) _____

13) _____

14) _____

15) _____

CHOICES

Bifurcate ligament
Dorsal calcaneocuboid ligaments
Dorsal cuboideonavicular ligament
Dorsal cuneocuboid ligament
Dorsal cuneonavicular ligaments
Dorsal intercuneiform ligaments
Long plantar ligament (2)
Navicular
Plantar calcaneocuboid
    (short plantar) ligament (2)
Plantar calcaneonavicular
    (spring) ligament (2)
Plantar cuboideonavicular ligament
Plantar metatarsal ligaments

Please answer the following questions.

1) The fibular collateral ligament spans between which two bony landmarks?

_____   _____

2) Both collateral ligaments resist which rotation of the tibia? _____

3) Aside from helping the femoral condyles sit upon the tibial plateaus, the menisci of the knee are also important

for _____ and _____.

4) To access the edge of the medial meniscus, you would slowly rotate the knee in which direction?

_____

5) The small, fluid-filled sac located directly superficial to the patella is the _____.

6) The common peroneal nerve lies _____ to the biceps femoris tendon and _____ to the

gastrocnemius belly. It becomes accessible along the _____ surface of the head of the fibula.

7) To feel the tension change in the plantar aponeurosis, what action could you passively perform at the foot?

_____

8) The deltoid ligament originates at the medial malleolus and fans distally out to which three bones/bony landmarks?

_____   _____   _____

9) The plantar calcaneonavicular (spring) ligament stretches from the _____ to

the _____ and may be deep to the _____.

10) The fibers of the extensor retinacula have two palpable distinctions from the extensor tendons. What are they?

_____   _____

11) The flexor retinaculum can be located between which two bony landmarks?

_____   _____

12) The posterior tibial artery can be located just _____ and _____ to the medial malleolus.

13) Between the first and second metatarsals of the foot you can feel the pulse of which artery?

_____

14) The calcaneal bursa is located between the attachment of the _____ and the _____.

Notes

Notes

Italicized page numbers after the answers indicate where the information can be found in *Trail Guide*.

 # Introduction

Tour Guide Tips #1, p. 1
1) bony landmarks - *p. 12*
2) Even though the topography, shape and proportion are unique, the body's composition and structures are virtually identical on all individuals. - *p. 12*
3) To examine or explore by touching (an organ or area of the body), usually as a diagnostic aid - *p. 14*
4) locating, aware, assessing - *p. 14*
5) directs movement, depth. - *p. 14*
6) • read the information
   • visualize what you are trying to access
   • verbalize to your partner what you feel
   • locate the structure first on yourself
   • read the text aloud
   • be patient - *p. 15*
7) across, along - *p. 16*
8) stay still - *p. 16*
9) active, passive - *p. 17*
10) lengths, shapes, edges - *p. 17*
11) • move slowly
    • avoid using excessive pressure
    • focus your awareness - be present - *p. 18*
12) muscle cells, layers of connective tissue - *p. 21*
13) tendon - *p. 21*

Tour Guide Tips #2, p. 2
1) prime mover, antagonist - *p. 21*
2) striated texture, direction of the muscle fibers, it can be in contracted or relaxed state - *p. 21, 22*
3) attachments, variable tension - *p. 23*
4) tendon, ligament, fascia, periosteum, retinaculum, aponeurosis, adipose - *p. 23-27*
5) fibrous membrane, skin - *p. 24*
6) compression or impingement of a nerve - *p. 27*

Matching
1) N   adipose - *p. 27*
2) F   aponeurosis - *p. 23*
3) D   artery - *p. 26*
4) H   bone - *p. 20*
5) E   bursa - *p. 26*
6) B   fascia - *p. 24*
7) G   ligament - *p. 23*
8) I   lymph node - *p. 27*
9) A   muscle - *p. 21*
10) J   nerve - *p. 27*
11) K   retinaculum - *p. 25*
12) L   skin - *p. 20*
13) M   tendon - *p. 23*
14) C   vein - *p. 26*

Exploring Texture #1, p. 3
1) epidermis
2) dermis
3) arrector pili muscle
4) sweat gland
5) hair follicle
6) blood vessels
7) muscle fibers
8) endomysium
9) perimysium
10) epimysium
11) bone
12) blood vessels
13) neurovascular bundle
14) tendon
15) periosteum

Types of Muscle Bellies & Joints, p. 4
1) bipennate
2) multibelly
3) unipennate
4) convergent
5) biceps
6) fusiform
7) gliding
8) hinge
9) ellipsoid
10) pivot
11) ball-and-socket
12) saddle

Exploring Texture #2, p. 5
1) muscle tissue
2) bone
3) periosteum
4) interosseous membrane
5) deep fascia
6) adipose (fatty) tissue
7) superficial fascia
8) skin
9) deep fascia

 # Navigating

Regions of Body, p. 6
1) pectoral
2) axillary
3) brachial
4) cubital
5) abdominal
6) inguinal
7) pubic
8) femoral
9) facial
10) mandibular
11) supraclavicular
12) antecubital
13) patellar
14) crural
15) cranial
16) cervical
17) scapular
18) thoracic
19) lumbar
20) pelvic
21) sural
22) gluteal
23) popliteal

Planes, Directions, Positions & Movements #1, p. 7
1) transverse
2) sagittal
3) frontal
4) superior
5) inferior
6) posterior
7) anterior
8) proximal
9) distal
10) medial
11) lateral
12) superficial
13) deep

Planes, Directions, Positions & Movements #2, p. 8
1) C   anterior
2) J   deep
3) B   distal
4) E   inferior
5) I   lateral
6) H   medial
7) A   posterior
8) G   proximal
9) F   superficial

10) D   superior
11) K   abduction
12) V   adduction
13) P   circumduction
14) T   dorsiflexion
15) U   extension
16) S   flexion
17) Q   lateral flexion
18) M   lateral rotation
19) L   medial rotation
20) O   plantar flexion
21) W   pronation
22) R   rotation
23) N   supination

Movements of the Body #1-5, p. 9-13
1) supination of forearm
2) depression of scapula
3) depression of mandible
4) abduction of hip
5) adduction of shoulder
6) flexion of wrist
7) flexion of thumb
8) inversion of foot
9) rotation of spine
10) upward rotation of scapula
11) posterior tilt (upward rotation) of pelvis
12) lateral deviation of mandible
13) adduction (ulnar deviation) of wrist
14) extension of fingers
15) anterior tilt (downward rotation) of pelvis
16) extension of elbow
17) extension of wrist
18) elevation of scapula
19) elevation of mandible
20) lateral flexion of spine
21) adduction of hip
22) extension of hip
23) abduction of shoulder
24) extension of neck
25) adduction (or retraction) of scapula
26) lateral flexion of neck
27) adduction of fingers
28) flexion of fingers
29) lateral tilt (elevation) of pelvis
30) abduction (or protraction) of scapula
31) lateral rotation of hip
32) flexion of hip
33) flexion of elbow
34) pronation of forearm
35) abduction of fingers
36) lateral rotation of shoulder

37) extension of spine
38) flexion of knee
39) flexion of neck
40) abduction of thumb
41) dorsiflexion of ankle
42) medial rotation of shoulder
43) extension of knee
44) horizontal adduction of shoulder
45) abduction (radial deviation) of wrist
46) eversion of foot
47) medial rotation of hip
48) protraction of mandible
49) opposition of thumb
50) retraction of mandible
51) extension of thumb
52) plantar flexion of ankle
53) flexion of spine
54) downward rotation of scapula
55) extension of shoulder
56) adduction of thumb
57) rotation of neck
58) flexion of shoulder
59) horizontal abduction of shoulder
60) elevation/expansion of ribs (inhalation)

Skeletal System #1, p. 14
1) ribs
2) lumbar vertebra
3) pelvis
4) sacrum
5) femur
6) patella
7) fibula
8) tibia
9) skull
10) mandible
11) cervical vertebra
12) clavicle
13) scapula
14) humerus
15) ulna
16) radius
17) carpals
18) phalanges
19) tarsals
20) metatarsals
21) phalanges
22) axial

Skeletal System #2, p. 15
1) skull
2) mandible
3) cervical vertebra
4) clavicle

5) scapula
6) thoracic vertebra
7) twelfth rib
8) lumbar vertebra
9) pelvis
10) sacrum
11) coccyx
12) humerus
13) radius
14) ulna
15) femur
16) tibia
17) fibula
18) talus
19) calcaneus
20) appendicular

Muscular System #1, p. 16
1) frontalis
2) platysma
3) deltoid
4) pectoralis major
5) biceps brachii
6) pronator teres
7) flexors of forearm
8) external oblique
9) rectus abdominis
10) adductors
11) sartorius
12) rectus femoris
13) vastus medialis
14) peroneus longus
15) tibialis anterior
16) sternocleidomastoid
17) pectoralis minor
18) coracobrachialis
19) brachialis
20) transverse abdominis
21) brachioradialis
22) flexor digitorum superficialis
23) vastus lateralis
24) vastus intermedius

Muscular System #2, p. 17
1) trapezius
2) deltoid
3) triceps brachii
4) latissimus dorsi
5) extensors of the forearm
6) gluteus maximus
7) iliotibial tract
8) biceps femoris
9) semitendinosus
10) gastrocnemius
11) temporalis

12) splenius capitis
13) levator scapula
14) supraspinatus
15) rhomboids
16) infraspinatus
17) teres minor
18) teres major
19) erector spinae group
20) long muscles of the thumb
21) gluteus minimus
22) semimembranosus
23) soleus

Muscular System #3, p. 18
1) sternocleidomastoid
2) trapezius
3) deltoid
4) teres major
5) latissimus dorsi
6) gluteus medius
7) gluteus maximus
8) vastus lateralis
9) biceps femoris
10) gastrocnemius
11) peroneus longus
12) soleus
13) temporalis
14) platysma
15) extensors of the forearm
16) biceps brachii
17) brachialis
18) triceps brachii
19) serratus anterior
20) rectus abdominis
21) external oblique
22) tensor fasciae latae
23) rectus femoris
24) vastus lateralis
25) iliotibial tract
26) tibialis anterior

Fascial System #1, p. 19
1) brachial fascia
2) biceps brachii
3) humerus
4) lateral intermuscular septum
5) triceps brachii
6) medial intermuscular septum
7) antebrachial fascia
8) flexor muscles
9) radius
10) ulna
11) interosseous membrane
12) extensor muscles

Fascial System #2, p. 20
1) lateral intermuscular septum
2) quadriceps
3) iliotibial tract
4) femur
5) fascia lata
6) medial intermuscular septum
7) adductors
8) hamstrings
9) tibia
10) interosseous membrane
11) deep crural fascia
12) crural fascia
13) fibula

Cardiovascular System - Arteries, p. 21
1) left and right common carotid
2) arch of aorta
3) ascending aorta
4) heart
5) abdominal aorta
6) right common iliac
7) femoral
8) popliteal
9) anterior tibial
10) posterior tibial
11) dorsalis pedis
12) dorsal arch
13) vertebral
14) brachiocephalic
15) subclavian
16) axillary
17) brachial
18) radial
19) ulnar

Cardiovascular System - Veins, p. 22
1) brachiocephalic
2) superior vena cava
3) heart
4) inferior vena cava
5) common iliac
6) femoral
7) great saphenous
8) internal jugular
9) external jugular
10) subclavian
11) axillary
12) cephalic
13) brachial
14) basilic
15) popliteal
16) peroneal
17) posterior tibial
18) anterior tibial

Nervous System, p. 23
1) brain
2) cervical plexus
3) brachial plexus
4) spinal cord
5) lumbar plexus
6) sacral plexus
7) sciatic
8) femoral
9) musculocutaneous
10) radial
11) median
12) ulnar
13) cauda equina
14) tibial
15) common peroneal

Lymphatic System, p. 24
1) cervical lymph nodes
2) thymus gland
3) axillary lymph nodes
4) lymphatic vessels
5) cisterna chyli
6) iliac lymph nodes
7) inguinal lymph nodes
8) lymphatic vessels
9) tonsils
10) internal jugular vein
11) subclavian vein
12) thoracic duct
13) spleen
14) aggregated lymphatic follicle (Peyer's patch)
15) bone marrow

Shoulder & Arm

Topographical Views, p. 25
1) superior nuchal line of the occiput
2) trapezius
3) spine of the scapula
4) inferior angle of the scapula
5) triceps brachii
6) latissimus dorsi
7) triceps brachii
8) deltoid
9) axilla
10) latissimus dorsi
11) serratus anterior
12) acromion
13) pectoralis major

14) deltoid
15) biceps brachii
16) trapezius
17) clavicle

Bones & Bony Landmarks #1, p. 26
1) clavicle, scapula, humerus - *p. 56*
2) synovial - *p. 56*
3) sternoclavicular - *p. 56*
4) glenohumeral - *p. 56*
5) spine of the scapula - *p. 60*
6) in the small of the back - *p. 61*
7) serratus anterior - *p. 61*
8) levator scapula, trapezius - *p. 61*
9) teres major and minor - *p. 62*
10) use your broad thumbpad - *p. 62*

Bones & Bony Landmarks #2, p. 27
1) infraspinatus, supraspinatus, subscapularis - *p. 63, 64*
2) spine of the scapula, medial border, lateral border - *p. 63*
3) acromion, clavicle - *p. 63*
4) maneuver partner's arm and scapula in a way which allows thumb to sink in further - *p. 64*
5) sidelying with your partner's arm lying against his side - *p. 64*
6) trapezius, deltoid - *p. 65*
7) acromial, sternal - *p. 65*
8) elevation, depression - *p. 66*
9) deltopectoral - *p. 67*
10) shape, size - *p. 67*
11) supraspinatus, infraspinatus and teres minor - *p. 68*
12) long head of the biceps brachii - *p. 68*

Extra Credit: 16
trapezius
levator scapula
supraspinatus
infraspinatus
subscapularis
teres minor
rhomboid major
rhomboid minor
biceps brachii
triceps brachii
coracobrachialis
pectoralis minor
omohyoid
deltoid
serratus anterior
teres major

Bones of Shoulder & Arm #1, p. 28
1) sternoclavicular (S/C) joint
2) clavicle
3) acromioclavicular (A/C) joint
4) glenohumeral joint
5) scapula
6) humerus
7) acromion
8) superior notch
9) coracoid process
10) superior angle
11) supraglenoid tubercle
12) glenoid cavity
13) infraglenoid tubercle
14) subscapular fossa
15) lateral border
16) medial border
17) inferior angle

Bones of Shoulder & Arm #2, p. 29
1) greater tubercle
2) deltoid tuberosity
3) lesser tubercle
4) intertubercular groove
5) head of humerus
6) greater tubercle
7) deltoid tuberosity
8) superior angle
9) supraspinous fossa
10) acromion
11) acromial angle
12) spine of the scapula
13) infraspinous fossa
14) lateral border
15) medial border
16) inferior angle

Muscles of Shoulder & Arm #1, p. 30
1) trapezius
2) deltoid
3) levator scapula
4) rhomboid minor
5) rhomboid major
6) supraspinatus
7) infraspinatus
8) teres minor
9) teres major
10) triceps brachii
11) erector spinae group
12) serratus posterior inferior
13) latissimus dorsi
14) thoracolumbar aponeurosis

Muscles of Shoulder & Arm #2, p. 31
1) levator scapula
2) trapezius
3) deltoid
4) infraspinatus
5) teres minor
6) teres major
7) latissimus dorsi
8) biceps brachii
9) brachialis
10) triceps brachii
11) serratus anterior
12) external oblique
13) trapezius
14) deltoid
15) pectoralis major
16) serratus anterior
17) biceps brachii
18) pectoralis minor
19) coracobrachialis
20) latissimus dorsi

Color the Muscles, p. 32 & 33

Muscles and Movements #1, p. 34
1) glenohumeral
2) horizontal adduction of shoulder
3) deltoid (anterior fibers)
   pectoralis major (upper fibers)
4) infraspinatus
5) adduction (retraction) of scapula
6) trapezius (middle fibers)
   rhomboid major
   rhomboid minor
7) pectoralis minor
8) lateral (external) rotation of the shoulder
9) deltoid (posterior fibers)
   teres minor
10) subscapularis

Muscles and Movements #2, p. 35
1) glenohumeral
2) adduction of the shoulder
3) infraspinatus
   teres major
   teres minor
   triceps brachii (long head)
4) supraspinatus
5) downward rotation of the scapula
6) rhomboid major
   rhomboid minor
   levator scapula
7) trapezius (upper and lower fibers)

8) abduction (protraction) of the scapula
9) serratus anterior (with origin fixed)
   pectoralis minor
10) rhomboid major
    rhomboid minor
11) horizontal abduction of the shoulder
12) infraspinatus
    teres minor
13) pectoralis major (upper fibers)

Muscles and Movements #3, p. 36
1) scapulothoracic
2) depression of the scapula
3) serratus anterior (with origin fixed)
   pectoralis minor
4) rhomboid major
   rhomboid minor
5) extension of the shoulder
6) deltoid (posterior fibers)
   latissimus dorsi
7) biceps brachii
8) abduction of the shoulder
9) deltoid (all fibers)
   supraspinatus
10) pectoralis major (all fibers)

Muscles and Movements #4, p. 37
1) glenohumeral
2) medial (internal) rotation
   of the shoulder
3) subscapularis
   pectoralis major (all fibers)
4) infraspinatus
5) elevation of scapula
6) rhomboid major
   rhomboid minor
   levator scapula
7) serratus anterior (with origin fixed)
8) flexion of the shoulder
9) biceps brachii
   coracobrachialis
10) latissimus dorsi
11) upward rotation of scapula
12) trapezius (upper and lower fibers)
13) rhomboid major
    rhomboid minor

What's the Muscle? p. 38
1) pectoralis major
2) teres major
3) rhomboid minor
4) coracobrachialis
5) infraspinatus

6) serratus anterior
7) levator scapula
8) trapezius
9) triceps brachii
10) supraspinatus
11) rhomboid major
12) teres minor
13) subscapularis
14) deltoid
15) pectoralis minor
16) latissimus dorsi

Muscle Group #1, p. 39
1) trapezius - p. 75
2) abduct the shoulder - p. 75
3) antagonist - p. 75-76
4) depress - p. 76
5) extension - p. 77
6) adduction (retraction) of scapula or "bring your shoulder up off the table" - p. 78
7) middle portion - p. 79
8) grasp tissue and let it slip through your fingers; feel for the muscle's fibrous texture - p. 80
9) lateral border of the scapula - p. 81

10) lengthen
11) shorten, lengthen
12) lengthen
13) shorten
14) shorten
15) lengthen
16) shorten
17) shorten

Muscle Group #1, p. 40

Muscle	O	I
deltoid	2	6
latissimus dorsi	4	5
teres major	3	5
trapezius	1	7

Muscle Group #2, p. 41
1) glenohumeral - p. 82
2) trapezius (upper fibers) - p. 82
3) supraspinatus - p. 82
4) thick, layered fascia - p. 82
5) subscapular fossa, serratus anterior - p. 82
6) abduction of the shoulder - p. 84
7) spine of the scapula, medial border, lateral border - p. 85
8) deltoid - p. 85

9) teres minor is smaller, teres major medially rotates the shoulder, teres minor laterally rotates the shoulder - p. 79, 82
10) latissimus dorsi and teres major - p. 86
11) medially rotate the shoulder - p. 86
12) deltoid - p. 87
13) flex the shoulder to 90°, then horizontally adduct and laterally rotate the shoulder 10° - p. 89
14) biceps brachii - p. 89
15) inferior and lateral - p. 89

Muscle Group #2, p. 42

Muscle	O	I
infraspinatus	1	5
subscapularis	2	6
supraspinatus	4	5
teres minor	3	5

7) lengthen
8) shorten
9) lengthen
10) lengthen

Muscle Group #3, p. 43
1) trapezius, erector spinae muscles - p. 90
2) adduct or elevate the scapula are two synergistic actions; the trapezius upwardly rotates the scapula, while the rhomboids downwardly rotate it - p. 90, 76 - 77
3) splenius capitis, posterior scalene - p. 92, 93
4) elevation of the scapula - p. 93
5) shifts the cervical TVPs further anterior, gives the levator more palpable tension and shortens and softens the overlying trapezius - p. 93
6) rhomboids - p. 94
7) latissimus dorsi or pectoralis major - p. 94
8) trapezius and rhomboids - p. 96
9) clavicular, sternal and costal - p. 97
10) *examples: giving a hug, doing a push-up, lifting a stack of heavy anatomy books*
11) communicating your intentions to your partner - p. 98
12) deltoid - p. 98

13) brings the pectoralis major off the chest wall, allows breast tissue to fall away - *p. 99*

14) brachial plexus, axillary artery and vein - *p. 100*

Muscle Group #3, p. 44

Muscle	O	I
levator scapula	7	12
pectoralis major	2	10
pectoralis minor	6	9
rhomboid major	4	13
rhomboid minor	3	14
serratus anterior	5	8
subclavius	1	11

Muscle Group #4, p. 45

1) long head - *p. 103*
2) *examples: turning a doorknob, tightening your gasoline cap, digging in the sand*
3) deltoid (anterior fibers) - *p. 103*
4) bicipital aponeurosis - *p. 104*
5) teres major and minor - *p. 105*
6) olecranon process - *p. 106*
7) extend his elbow (against your resistance) - *p. 106*
8) pectoralis major and anterior deltoid - *p. 107*
9) laterally rotate and abduct the shoulder to 45° - *p. 107*
10) pectoralis major - *p. 107*

11) lengthen
12) lengthen
13) lengthen
14) lengthen

Muscle Group #4, p. 46

Muscle	O	I
biceps brachii	2	6
coracobrachialis	1	4
triceps brachii	3	5

Other Structures, p. 47

1) acromioclavicular ligament
2) acromion
3) coracoacromial ligament
4) coracohumeral ligament
5) biceps brachii tendon (cut)
6) coracoclavicular ligament
7) trapezoid
8) conoid
9) coracoid process
10) glenohumeral joint capsule

Fill In

11) immediately release and adjust your position posteriorly - *p. 109*
12) clavicle, coracoid process - *p. 112*
13) coracoacromial - *p. 112*
14) extend - *p. 112*
15) extend the shoulder - *p. 113*
16) biceps brachii and triceps brachii - *p. 114*

Glenohumeral Joint #1, p. 48

1) acromion
2) supraspinatus tendon
3) subacromial bursa
4) infraspinatus tendon
5) glenoid cavity
6) teres minor tendon
7) synovial membrane
8) coracoid process
9) superior glenohumeral ligament
10) biceps brachii tendon (long head)
11) subscapularis tendon
12) middle glenohumeral ligament
13) inferior glenohumeral ligament

Glenohumeral Joint #2, p. 49

1) acromioclavicular joint and ligament
2) supraspinatus tendon
3) acromion
4) subacromial bursa
5) deltoid
6) capsular ligament
7) synovial membrane
8) glenoid labrum
9) cartilage of glenoid cavity
10) articular capsule

Sternoclavicular Joint, p. 50

1) clavicle
2) anterior sternoclavicular ligament
3) first rib
4) costal cartilages
5) second rib
6) radiate sternocostal ligament
7) interclavicular ligament
8) articular disc
9) joint cavity
10) costoclavicular ligament
11) sternocostal synchondrosis
12) manubrium
13) sternocostal joints

Forearm & Hand

Topographical Views, p. 52

1) brachioradialis
2) extensor crease of the wrist
3) metacarpophalangeal joints
4) lateral epicondyle
5) olecranon process
6) extensor muscles
7) shaft of the ulna
8) head of the ulna
9) extensor digitorum tendons
10) biceps brachii tendon
11) brachioradialis
12) thenar eminence
13) medial epicondyle
14) flexor muscles
15) flexor carpi radialis tendon
16) palmaris longus tendon
17) flexor carpi ulnaris tendon
18) flexor crease of the wrist
19) hypothenar eminence

Bones & Bony Landmarks, p. 53

1) ulna - *p. 118*
2) pronation, supination - *p. 118*
3) humeroulnar, humeroradial - *p. 118*
4) "flexor crease" - *p. 118*
5) triceps brachii - *p. 122*
6) lateral epicondyle - *p. 122*
7) head of the ulna - *p. 124*
8) annular - *p. 125*
9) styloid process - *p. 126*
10) head of the ulna - *p. 126*
11) carpals - *p. 126*

Humerus, p. 54

1) greater tubercle
2) deltoid tuberosity
3) lateral supracondylar ridge
4) lateral epicondyle
5) head of humerus
6) lesser tubercle
7) intertubercular groove
8) medial supracondylar ridge
9) medial epicondyle
10) head of humerus
11) medial supracondylar ridge
12) medial epicondyle
13) greater tubercle
14) deltoid tuberosity
15) lateral supracondylar ridge
16) olecranon fossa
17) lateral epicondyle

Radius & Ulna, p. 55

1) carpals
2) metacarpals
3) ulna
4) radius
5) phalanges
6) head of the radius
7) radial tuberosity
8) styloid process of the radius
9) olecranon process
10) coronoid process
11) shaft of the ulna
12) styloid process of the ulna
13) olecranon process
14) head of the radius
15) shaft of the radius
16) Lister's tubercle
17) styloid process of the radius

Carpals, p. 56

1) scaphoid
2) lunate
3) triquetrum
4) pisiform
5) scaphoid tubercle
6) trapezium tubercle
7) trapezium
8) trapezoid
9) capitate
10) hook of the hamate
11) hamate
12) lunate
13) scaphoid
14) pisiform
15) triquetrum
16) hamate
17) capitate
18) trapezoid
19) trapezium

**Bones & Bony Landmarks of
Wrist & Hand #1, p. 57**

1) palmar, dorsal, radial, ulnar - *p. 128*
2) flexor crease of the wrist - *p. 128*
3) pisiform - *p. 129*
4) flexor carpi ulnaris - *p. 129*
5) triquetrum - *p. 129*
6) hamate - *p. 130*
7) flexor retinaculum - *p. 130*
8) ulnar artery, ulnar nerve - *p. 130*
9) pisiform, (hook of the) hamate, scaphoid (tubercle), trapezium (tubercle) - *p. 130, 132*
10) scaphoid - *p. 131*

11) trapezium - *p. 131*
12) scaphoid - *p. 131*
13) lunate, capitate - *p. 133*
14) metacarpophalangeal - *p. 134*

Extra Credit - *p. 127*

scaphoid
lunate
triquetrum
pisiform
trapezium
trapezoid
capitate
hamate

(pneumonic example beginning with proximal row of carpals:
Some **L**overs **T**ry **P**ositions
That **T**hey **C**an't **H**andle)

**Bones & Bony Landmarks of
Wrist & Hand #2, p. 58**

1) metacarpals
2) base
3) shaft
4) head
5) base
6) shaft
7) head
8) phalanges
9) proximal phalange
10) middle phalange
11) distal phalange

Muscles of Forearm #1, p. 59

1) brachioradialis
2) flexor pollicis longus
3) biceps brachii
4) brachialis
5) pronator teres
6) bicipital aponeurosis
7) flexor carpi radialis
8) palmaris longus
9) flexor carpi ulnaris
10) flexor digitorum superficialis
11) antebrachial fascia
12) palmar aponeurosis

Muscles of Forearm #2, p. 60

1) anconeus
2) extensor carpi ulnaris
3) extensor digitorum
4) extensor digiti minimi
5) extensor indicis

6) brachioradialis
7) extensor carpi radialis longus
8) extensor carpi radialis brevis
9) abductor pollicis longus
10) extensor pollicis brevis
11) extensor pollicis longus

Color the Muscles #1-2, p. 61 & 62

Muscles and Movements #1, p. 63

1) proximal and distal radioulnar joints
2) supination of forearm
3) biceps brachii
   brachioradialis (assists)
   supinator
4) pronator teres
   pronator quadratus
5) adduction of fingers
6) palmar interossei
7) abduction of thumb
8) abductor pollicis longus
   abductor pollicis brevis
9) adductor pollicis
10) flexion of elbow
11) flexor carpi radialis
   flexor carpi ulnaris (assists)
   palmaris longus
   pronator teres (assists)
12) triceps brachii (all heads)

Muscles and Movements #2, p. 64

1) radiocarpal
2) abduction (radial deviation) of wrist
3) extensor carpi radialis longus
   extensor carpi radialis brevis
   flexor carpi radialis
4) extensor carpi ulnaris
5) extension of thumb
6) extensor pollicis longus
   extensor pollicis brevis
   abductor pollicis longus
7) flexor pollicis longus
   flexor pollicis brevis
8) pronation of the forearm
9) pronator teres
   pronator quadratus
   brachioradialis (assists)
10) biceps brachii
   brachioradialis (assists)
11) abduction of fingers
12) dorsal interossei

Muscles and Movements #3, p. 65

1) first carpometacarpal
2) adduction of thumb
3) adductor pollicis
   palmar interossei (first)
4) abductor pollicis longus
   abductor pollicis brevis
5) opposition of thumb
6) opponens pollicis
   flexor pollicis brevis (assists)
7) flexion of wrist
8) flexor carpi radialis
   flexor carpi ulnaris
   flexor digitorum superficialis
   flexor digitorum profundus (assists)
9) extensor carpi radialis longus
   extensor carpi radialis brevis
   extensor carpi ulnaris
   extensor digitorum (assists)
10) adduction (ulnar deviation)
   of wrist
11) extensor carpi ulnaris
   flexor carpi ulnaris
12) flexor carpi radialis

Muscles and Movements #4, p. 66

1) humeroulnar, humeroradial
2) extension of elbow
3) triceps brachii (all heads)
   anconeus
4) biceps brachii
   brachialis
   brachioradialis
5) flexion of thumb
6) flexor pollicis longus
   flexor pollicis brevis
   adductor pollicis (assists)
7) abductor pollicis longus
8) extension of wrist
9) extensor carpi radialis longus
   extensor carpi radialis brevis
   extensor carpi ulnaris
   extensor digitorum (assists)
10) palmaris longus

What's the Muscle? #1, p. 67

1) flexor carpi radialis
2) extensor carpi ulnaris
3) extensor carpi radialis longus
4) brachioradialis
5) supinator
6) palmaris longus
7) flexor digitorum profundus
8) opponens pollicis

What's the Muscle? #2, p. 68

1) flexor digitorum superficialis
2) adductor pollicis
3) extensor carpi radialis brevis
4) pronator teres
5) flexor carpi ulnaris
6) brachialis
7) extensor digitorum

Muscle Group #1, p. 69

1) brachialis - p. 140
2) flexors, extensors - p. 141
3) brachioradialis - p. 141
4) flexor, lateral - p. 155
5) pronator teres - p. 154
6) biceps brachii - p. 154
7) extensors - p. 155

8) lengthen
9) shorten
10) lengthen
11) shorten

Fill In

12) pronator teres
13) brachialis
14) pronator quadratus
15) brachioradialis
16) supinator

Muscle Group #1, p. 70

Muscle	O	I
brachialis	1	10
brachioradialis	2	9
pronator quadratus	3	6
pronator teres	4	8
supinator	5	7

Muscle Group #2, p. 71

1) extensor, flexor - p. 142
2) shaft of the ulna - p. 142
3) • it's a **flexor**
   • there must be an **extensor** carpi radialis
   • it extends the **carpals** (crosses the wrist joint)
   • there's a muscle that flexes the **digits**
   • on the **radial** side of forearm
   • must be a flexor carpi **ulnaris**
   - p. 137

4) extensor carpi ulnaris - p. 143
5) second through fifth - p. 144
6) extensor, flexor - p. 142, 143
7) brachioradialis, extensor carpi radialis longus and brevis - p. 146
8) abduct - p. 145
9) flexor carpi radialis, palmaris longus and flexor carpi ulnaris - p. 148
10) four, carpal tunnel - p. 148
11) palmaris longus - p. 151
12) flexor carpi ulnaris - p. 152
13) ulnar shaft - p. 153

Muscle Group #2, p. 72

Muscle	O	I
extensor carpi radialis brevis	5	9
extensor carpi radialis longus	5	8
extensor carpi ulnaris	2	6
extensor digitorum	2	13
flexor carpi radialis	3	7
flexor carpi ulnaris	3	14
flexor digitorum profundus	1	10
flexor digitorum superficialis	4	11
palmaris longus	3	12

15) shorten
16) lengthen
17) shorten
18) lengthen
19) lengthen

Muscle Group #3, p. 73

1) thenar, hypothenar - p. 165
2) eight, four - p. 157
3) opponens pollicis - p. 157
4) abductor pollicis, extensor pollicis longus and brevis - p. 160, 162
5) lumbricals, metacarpals - p. 163
6) flexor digitorum profundus - p. 163
7) abductor digiti minimi - p. 165

What's the Muscle?

8) adductor pollicis
9) palmar interossei
10) lumbricals
11) dorsal interossei

208

Muscle Group #3, p. 74

Muscle	O	I
abductor pollicis longus	4	6
adductor pollicis	2	7
extensor pollicis longus	5	8
flexor pollicis longus	1	8
opponens pollicis	3	9

Other Structures, p. 75

1) radial and ulnar collateral ligaments - *p. 166, 167*
2) annular ligament - *p. 167*
3) medial epicondyle and olecranon process - *p. 167*
4) olecranon bursa - *p. 168*
5) flexor tendons, median - *p. 169*
6) flexor retinaculum - *p. 169*
7) palmar aponeurosis - *p. 169*
8) radial - *p. 170*

Fill In

9) flexor retinaculum
10) antebrachial fascia
11) median nerve
12) carpals
13) carpal tunnel

Humeroulnar & Proximal Radioulnar Joints, p. 76

1) humerus
2) head of radius (deep)
3) annular ligament
4) radius
5) ulna
6) radial collateral ligament
7) articular capsule
8) radius
9) annular ligament
10) articular capsule
11) humerus
12) medial epicondyle
13) ulnar collateral ligament
14) olecranon process
15) ulna

Radiocarpal Joint, p. 77

1) palmar radiocarpal ligament
2) radioscapholunate part
3) radiotriquetral part
4) radiocapitate part
5) palmar radioulnar ligament
6) palmar ulnocarpal ligament
7) ulnolunate part
8) ulnotriquetral part

9) ulnar collateral ligament
10) dorsal radioulnar ligament
11) dorsal radiocarpal ligament
12) radial collateral ligament

Intercarpal Joints & more, p. 78

1) palmar intercarpal ligaments
2) radiate carpal ligaments
3) pisohamate ligament
4) dorsal intercarpal ligaments
5) distal intercarpal ligaments
6) palmar carpometacarpal ligaments
7) palmar metacarpal ligaments
8) pisometacarpal ligament
9) dorsal carpometacarpal ligaments
10) dorsal metacarpal ligaments

Spine & Thorax

Topographical Views, p. 80

1) jugular notch
2) sternum
3) ribs
4) edge of rib cage
5) rectus abdominis
6) external oblique
7) umbilicus
8) iliac crest
9) medial border of the scapula
10) erector spinae group
11) twelfth rib
12) iliac crest
13) spinous process of C-7
14) spinous processes of thoracic and lumbar vertebrae
15) posterior superior iliac spine (PSIS)
16) sacrum

Bones & Bony Landmarks #1, p. 81

1) cervical - *p. 176*
2) sternum and rib cage - *p. 176*
3) spinous processes - *p. 182*
4) D   T-12
   C   T-2
   A   L-4
   B   C-7
   E   T-7   - *p. 180*
5) flexion, extension - *p. 182*
6) body type, muscular contraction - *p. 184*
7) C-2, C-7 - *p. 184, 185*
8) ligamentum nuchae - *p. 182*

9) sternocleidomastoid - *p.186*
10) mastoid process, center of shaft of clavicle - *p. 186*
11) spinous and transverse processes - *p. 187*

Bones & Bony Landmarks #2, p. 82

1) erector spinae, connecting aspects of the ribs - *p. 188*
2) two inches - *p. 188*
3) second - *p. 190*
4) costal cartilage - *p. 191*
5) intercostals - *p. 191*
6) the sides of the trunk - *p. 191*
7) clavicle - *p. 192*
8) scalenes - *p. 192*
9) slow, deep breath into upper chest - *p. 192*
10) anterior/posterior, lateral, superior - *p. 193*
11) 45 degrees - *p. 193*
12) erector spinae group - *p. 193*

Bones of Spine & Thorax, p. 83

1) cervical vertebra
2) ribs
3) thoracic vertebra
4) lumbar vertebra
5) sacrum
6) coccyx
7) manubrium
8) sternum
9) costal cartilage
10) lumbar vertebra
11) cervical spine, seven, lordotic
12) thoracic spine, twelve, kyphotic
13) lumbar spine, five, lordotic

First & Second Cervical Vertebrae, p. 84

1) posterior tubercle
2) transverse process
3) lamina
4) superior facets
5) articular facet for odontoid process
6) transverse process
7) lamina
8) vertebral foramen
9) groove for vertebral artery
10) transverse foramen
11) atlas
12) spinous process
13) vertebral foramen
14) odontoid process
15) transverse process

16) transverse foramen
17) lamina
18) axis
19) superior facets
20) odontoid process
21) lamina
22) spinous process
23) vertebral foramen
24) transverse process

Cervical Vertebrae, p. 85
1) posterior tubercle
2) anterior tubercle
3) canal for spinal nerve
4) transverse process
5) spinous process
6) transverse foramen
7) body
8) anterior tubercle
9) canal for spinal nerve
10) posterior tubercle
11) lamina groove
12) spinous process
13) lamina
14) superior facet
15) transverse process

Thoracic & Lumbar Vertebrae, p. 86
1) transverse process
2) superior facet
3) body
4) costal facets
5) spinous process
6) vertebral foramen
7) transverse process
8) lamina
9) spinous process
10) body
11) superior facet
12) lamina groove
13) spinous process
14) transverse process
15) body
16) transverse process
17) vertebral foramen
18) spinous process
19) body
20) superior facet
21) lamina groove

Rib Cage & Sternum, p. 87
1) first rib
2) second rib
3) sternocostal joint
4) costochondral joint

5) sternum
6) costal cartilage
7) true ribs (1-7)
8) false ribs (8-12)
9) floating ribs (11-12)
10) jugular notch
11) manubrium
12) sternal angle
13) body of sternum
14) articulations with ribs
15) xiphoid process

Muscles of Spine & Thorax #1, p. 88
1) splenius capitis
2) sternocleidomastoid
3) trapezius
4) deltoid
5) triceps brachii
6) latissimus dorsi
7) external oblique
8) thoracolumbar aponeurosis
9) semispinalis capitis
10) splenius capitis
11) splenius cervicis
12) levator scapula
13) supraspinatus
14) rhomboids
15) infraspinatus
16) teres minor
17) teres major
18) erector spinae group
19) serratus posterior inferior
20) external oblique
21) internal oblique

Muscles of Spine & Thorax #2, p. 89
1) semispinalis capitis
2) splenius capitis
3) serratus posterior superior
4) iliocostalis
5) longissimus thoracis
6) spinalis thoracis
7) serratus posterior inferior
8) internal oblique
9) rectus capitis posterior minor
10) oblique capitis superior
11) rectus capitis posterior major
12) oblique capitis inferior
13) longissimus capitis
14) spinalis cervicis
15) iliocostalis
16) longissimus thoracis
17) spinalis thoracis
18) transverse abdominis
19) thoracolumbar aponeurosis

Muscles of Spine & Thorax #3, p. 90
1) semispinalis capitis
2) splenius capitis
3) levator scapula
4) ligamentum nuchae
5) splenius cervicis
6) longissimus capitis
7) semispinalis capitis
8) splenius cervicis
9) semispinalis capitis
10) multifidi
11) rotatores

Cross Section of Neck, p. 91
1) sternocleidomastoid
2) anterior scalene
3) middle scalene
4) posterior scalene
5) levator scapula
6) trapezius
7) multifidi and spinalis cervicis
8) semispinalis cervicis
9) longissimus cervicis
10) longissimus capitis
11) splenius cervicis
12) semispinalis capitis
13) splenius capitis

Cross Section of Thorax #1, p. 92
1) intercostals
2) lung
3) iliocostalis
4) longissimus
5) multifidi and rotatores
6) trapezius
7) abdominal aorta
8) heart

Cross Section of Thorax #2, p. 93
1) rectus abdominis
2) external oblique
3) internal oblique
4) transverse abdominis
5) body of L-3
6) intestines
7) psoas minor
8) psoas major
9) quadratus lumborum
10) erector spinae group

Color the Muscles #1-4, p. 94-97

Muscles and Movements #1, p. 98

1) rotation of spine (vertebral column)
2) external oblique, his left
   internal oblique, his right
3) multifidi, his right
4) extension of spine
   (vertebral column)
5) spinalis (bilaterally)
   semispinalis capitis
   iliocostalis (bilaterally)
   intertransversarii (bilaterally)
   interspinalis
6) rectus abdominis
7) depression/collapse (exhalation)
   of ribs
8) internal intercostals (assists)
   serratus posterior inferior
9) external intercostals (assists)

Muscles and Movements #2, p. 99

1) flexion of spine (vertebral column)
2) external oblique (bilaterally)
   internal oblique (bilaterally)
3) quadratus lumborum (assists)
4) elevation/expansion (inhalation)
   of ribs
5) scalenes - anterior, middle, posterior
   sternocleidomastoid (assists)
   serratus posterior superior
   serratus anterior (if scapula is fixed)
   subclavius (first rib)
6) internal intercostals (assists)
7) lateral flexion of spine
   (vertebral column)
8) quadratus lumborum, his right
   external oblique, his right
9) spinalis, his left

What's the Muscle? #1, p. 100

1) rectus abdominis
2) rectus capitis posterior major
3) splenius cervicis
4) oblique capitis inferior
5) quadratus lumborum
6) longissimus
7) multifidi
8) splenius capitis

What's the Muscle? #2, p. 101

1) oblique capitis superior
2) iliocostalis
3) external oblique
4) semispinalis capitis

5) rectus capitis posterior minor
6) diaphragm
7) spinalis
8) rotatores

Muscle Group #1, p. 102

1) spinalis, iliocostalis - p. 202,
   illustration 4.49
2) thoracolumbar aponeurosis - p. 202
3) raise and lower his feet slightly
   - p. 205
4) trapezius, rhomboids or serratus
   posterior superior - p. 205
5) short, diagonal - p. 206
6) lamina groove - p. 206

Fill In

7) longissimus capitis
8) longissimus cervicis
9) longissimus thoracis
10) iliocostalis cervicis
11) iliocostalis thoracis
12) iliocostalis lumborum
13) spinalis cervicis
14) spinalis thoracis

Muscle Group #1, p. 103

Muscle	O	I
iliocostalis	1	12
longissimus	2	7
multifidi	3	9
rotatores	5	8
semispinalis capitis	6	11
spinalis	4	10

13) lengthen
14) shorten
15) shorten
16) lengthen

Muscle Group #2, p. 104

1) left - p. 209
2) trapezius, SCM - p. 209
3) rotate his head slightly toward the
   side you are palpating - p. 210
4) the trap's lateral edge is the same
   width as the suboccipitals - p. 211
5) spinous process of C-2, TVPs of
   C-1, the space between the superior nuchal line of the occiput and
   C-2 - p. 211

Draw the muscle

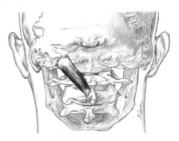

1) rectus capitis posterior major, p. 211

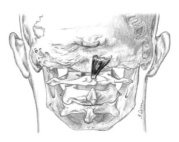

2) rectus capitis posterior minor, p. 211

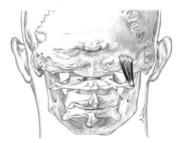

3) oblique capitis superior, p. 211

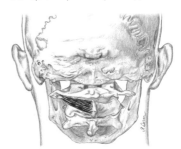

4) oblique capitis inferior, p. 211

Muscle Group #2, p. 105

Muscle	O	I
oblique capitis inferior	2	9
oblique capitis superior	4	6
rectus capitis post. major	2	7
rectus capitis post. minor	5	7
splenius capitis	1	8
splenius cervicis	3	10

11) shorten
12) shorten
13) shorten
14) lengthen
15) lengthen

Muscle Group #3, p. 106

1) lateral edge (side) - *p. 213*
2) twelfth rib, posterior iliac crest, transverse processes of lumbar vertebrae - *p. 214*
3) laterally tilt (elevate) the hip - *p. 214*
4) rectus abdominis - *p. 215, 216*
5) right - *p. 217*
6) external oblique - *p. 218*
7) diaphragm - *p. 219*
8) the central tendon - *p. 219*
9) only as your partner exhales - *p. 220*
10) latissimus dorsi, pectoralis major or external oblique - *p. 221*

Fill In

11) serratus anterior
12) external oblique
13) abdominal aponeurosis
14) inguinal ligament
15) rectus abdominis
16) linea alba
17) pubic crest
18) pubic symphysis

Muscle Group #3, p. 107

Muscle	O	I
diaphragm	1	10
external oblique	4	8
internal oblique	2	11
quadratus lumborum	5	12
rectus abdominis	6	9
transverse abdominis	3	7

13) shorten
14) lengthen
15) shorten
16) shorten
17) lengthen

Other Structures, p. 108

1) external occipital protuberance, spinous process of C-7 - *p. 224*
2) flexion and extension - *p. 224*
3) supraspinous - *p. 225*
4) medial - *p. 225*
5) latissimus dorsi, any branches of the erector spinae group - *p. 226*

Craniovertebral Joints #1, p. 109

1) basilar portion of occiput
2) capsule of atlantooccipital joint
3) atlas (C-1)
4) capsule of lateral atlantoaxial joint
5) axis (C-2)
6) capsule of zygapophyseal (lateral) joint
7) anterior longitudinal ligament
8) alar ligaments
9) cruciform ligament
10) superior longitudinal fibers
11) transverse ligament of atlas
12) inferior longitudinal fibers
13) atlas (C-1)
14) axis (C-2)

Craniovertebral Joints #2, p. 110

1) ligamentum nuchae
2) posterior atlantooccipital membrane
3) superior longitudinal fibers of cruciform ligament
4) occiput
5) atlas (C-1)
6) posterior atlantoaxial membrane
7) posterior longitudinal ligament
8) apical ligament
9) odontoid process of axis
10) anterior tubercle of atlas
11) transverse ligament of atlas
12) anterior longitudinal ligament
13) odontoid process of axis
14) synovial cavities
15) alar ligament
16) atlas (C-1)
17) transverse ligament of atlas

Intervertebral Joints, p. 111

1) body of vertebra
2) pedicle (cut)
3) posterior longitudinal ligament
4) posterior surface of vertebral body
5) intervertebral disc
6) pedicle (cut)
7) transverse process
8) ligamentum flavum
9) superior articular process
10) lamina
11) inferior articular facet

Costovertebral & Intervertebral Joints, p. 112

1) intervertebral disc (cut)
2) body of vertebra
3) synovial cavities
4) interarticular ligament
5) radiate ligament
6) superior costotransverse ligament (cut)
7) costotransverse ligament
8) lateral costotransverse ligament
9) anterior longitudinal ligament
10) transverse process
11) supraspinous ligament
12) spinous process
13) interspinous ligament
14) intervertebral foramen
15) ligamentum flavum
16) intervertebral disc
17) body of vertebra
18) posterior longitudinal ligament

Costovertebral & Sternocostal Joints, p. 113

1) transverse process
2) ligamentum flavum
3) radiate ligaments
4) lateral costotransverse ligament
5) superior costotransverse ligament
6) rib (cut)
7) interclavicular ligament
8) articular disc
9) clavicle
10) sternomanubrial joint
11) ribs
12) radiate ligaments
13) costoxiphoid ligament
14) costoclavicular ligament
15) sternocostal joints
16) costal cartilages
17) xiphoid process

Head, Neck & Face

Topographical View, p. 115
1) temporalis
2) zygomatic arch
3) condyle of the mandible
4) masseter
5) sternocleidomastoid
6) edge of trapezius
7) scalenes
8) clavicle
9) base of the mandible
10) hyoid bone
11) thyroid cartilage
12) jugular notch

Bones & Bony Landmarks, p. 116
1) SCM, base of the mandible, trachea - *p. 232*
2) posterior triangle - *p. 232*
3) twenty-two - *p. 234*
4) fibrous - *p. 234*
5) occiput - *p. 237*
6) external occipital protuberance - *p. 237*
7) superior nuchal line - *p. 237*
8) parietal - *p. 238*
9) mastoid process - *p. 239*
10) temporalis - *p. 239*
11) frontal - *p. 240*
12) submandibular fossa - *p. 241*
13) submandibular fossa - *p. 241*

Skull #1, p. 117
1) frontal
2) parietal
3) sphenoid
4) temporal
5) nasal
6) ethmoid
7) lacrimal
8) zygomatic
9) vomer
10) maxilla
11) mandible
12) sagittal suture
13) parietal
14) lambdoid suture
15) occiput
16) superior nuchal line
17) external occipital protuberance
18) mastoid process
19) maxilla
20) mandible

Skull #2, p. 118
1) occiput
2) parietal
3) temporal
4) frontal
5) sphenoid
6) ethmoid
7) lacrimal
8) nasal
9) zygomatic
10) maxilla
11) mandible
12) external occipital protuberance
13) temporal lines
14) external auditory meatus
15) mastoid process
16) condyle of the mandible
17) styloid process
18) temporomandibular joint
19) zygomatic arch
20) coronoid process
21) occiput
22) temporal
23) sphenoid
24) zygomatic
25) maxilla
26) palatine
27) vomer
28) mastoid process
29) foramen magnum
30) inferior nuchal line
31) superior nuchal line
32) external occipital protuberance

Mandible & Hyoid, p. 119
1) condyle
2) coronoid process
3) head
4) pterygoid fossa
5) neck
6) ramus
7) angle
8) body
9) mental foramen
10) base
11) greater horn
12) lesser horn
13) body

Temporomandibular Joint, p. 120
1) joint capsule
2) sphenomandibular ligament
3) lateral temporomandibular ligament
4) zygomatic arch

5) external auditory meatus
6) mastoid process
7) styloid process
8) stylomandibular ligament
9) mandible
10) articular disc of temporomandibular joint
11) lateral pterygoid
12) joint capsule
13) condyle of mandible (cut)
14) mandible
15) sphenomandibular ligament

Muscles of Head, Neck & Face #1, p. 121
1) galea aponeurotica
2) temporalis
3) occipitalis
4) digastric (posterior belly)
5) stylohyoid
6) splenius capitis
7) levator scapula
8) trapezius
9) posterior scalene
10) middle scalene
11) anterior scalene
12) omohyoid (inferior belly)
13) frontalis
14) masseter
15) digastric (anterior belly)
16) thyrohyoid
17) omohyoid (superior belly)
18) sternohyoid
19) sternothyroid
20) sternocleidomastoid

Muscles of Head, Neck & Face #2, p. 122
1) stylohyoid
2) digastric
3) internal jugular vein
4) common carotid artery
5) thyroid cartilage
6) omohyoid (cut)
7) sternothyroid (cut)
8) sternohyoid (cut)
9) mylohyoid
10) submandibular gland
11) thyrohyoid
12) omohyoid (superior belly)
13) sternohyoid
14) scalenes
15) trapezius
16) omohyoid (inferior belly)
17) sternocleidomastoid

Muscles of Face, p. 123
1) frontalis
2) procerus
3) corrugator supercili
4) orbicularis oculi
5) nasalis
6) levator labii superioris
7) zygomaticus major and minor
8) orbicularis oris
9) depressor anguli oris
10) mentalis
11) platysma

Color the Muscles #1-3, p. 124-126

Muscles and Movements #1, p. 127
1) protraction of mandible
2) lateral pterygoid (bilaterally)
   medial pterygoid (bilaterally)
3) temporalis
   digastric
4) extension of neck
   (cervical spine)
5) splenius capitis (bilaterally)
   splenius cervicis (bilaterally)
   semispinalis capitis
6) sternocleidomastoid (bilaterally)
   scalene, anterior (bilaterally)
7) flexion of neck (cervical spine)
8) longus capitis (bilaterally)
   longus colli (bilaterally)
9) levator scapula (bilaterally)
   longissimus capitis (assists)
   longissimus cervicis (assists)

Muscles and Movements #2, p. 128
1) depression of mandible
2) geniohyoid
   digastric (with hyoid bone fixed)
3) temporalis
4) rotation of neck
   (cervical spine)
5) middle scalene, his left
   trapezius (upper fibers), his left
6) levator scapula, his left
   longus colli, his left
   longus capitis, his left
   longissimus capitis, his left (assists)
   longissimus cervicis, his left (assists)
7) retraction of mandible
8) temporalis
   digastric
9) lateral pterygoid

Muscles and Movements #3, p. 129
1) temporomandibular
2) elevation of mandible
3) temporalis
   masseter
   medial pterygoid
4) geniohyoid
5) lateral flexion of neck
   (cervical spine)
6) splenius capitis
   splenius cervicis
   sternocleidomastoid
   scalenes - anterior, middle, posterior
   (with ribs fixed)

What's the Muscle? #1, p. 130
1) temporalis
2) sternothyroid
3) sternocleidomastoid
4) anterior scalene
5) stylohyoid
6) longus colli
7) medial pterygoid
8) posterior scalene
9) occipitofrontalis

What's the Muscle? #2, p. 131
1) longus capitis
2) middle scalene
3) platysma
4) masseter
5) omohyoid
6) lateral pterygoid
7) mylohyoid
8) sternohyoid
9) digastric

Muscle Group #1, p. 132
1) top of manubrium, medial 1/3
   of clavicle - *p. 250*
2) rotate head slightly to opposite
   side - *p. 251*
3) posterior - *p. 252*
4) scalenes - *p. 252*
5) anterior scalene, middle scalene
   - *p. 252*
6) scalenes - *p. 254*
7) sternocleidomastoid - *p. 254*
8) elevate the scapula - *p. 255*
9) masseter - *p. 256*
10) temporalis - *p. 257*
11) open your (mouth) jaw to access
    the coronoid process - *p. 258*

12) lengthen
13) shorten
14) shorten
15) shorten
16) lengthen
17) shorten

Muscle Group #1, p. 133
Muscle	O	I
anterior scalene	5	9
masseter	6	7
middle scalene	4	9
posterior scalene	3	11
sternocleidomastoid	2	10
temporalis	1	8

Muscle Group #2, p. 134
1) digastric, geniohyoid, mylohyoid,
   stylohyoid - *p. 259*
2) digastric - *p. 259*
3) press the tip of the tongue firmly
   against the roof of the mouth
   - *p. 260*
4) omohyoid - *p. 261*
5) platysma - *p. 263*
6) occipitalis, frontalis - *p. 263*
7) raise his eyebrows - *p. 264*
8) longus capitis and colli - *p. 266*

Muscle Group #2, p. 135
Muscle	O	I
digastric	2	7
geniohyoid	5	6
mylohyoid	5	6
omohyoid	4	6
sternohyoid	1	6
sternothyroid	1	8
stylohyoid	3	6

9) shorten
10) shorten
11) lengthen
12) shorten
13) lengthen

Other Structures, p. 136
1) temporal artery
2) facial nerve
3) external auditory meatus
4) parotid gland
5) common carotid artery
6) parotid duct
7) facial artery
8) submandibular gland

9) thyroid cartilage
10) cricoid cartilage
11) thyroid gland
12) trachea

Fill In

13) common carotid artery - *p. 268*
14) in front of the ear along the zygomatic arch - *p. 268*
15) facial artery - *p. 268*
16) jugular notch, cricoid ring - *p. 270*

 Pelvis & Thigh

Topographical Views, p. 137

1) rectus abdominis
2) iliac crest
3) anterior superior iliac spine (ASIS)
4) inguinal ligament
5) pubic crest
6) adductors
7) sartorius
8) rectus femoris
9) vastus medialis
10) patella
11) gluteus medius
12) greater trochanter
13) vastus lateralis
14) iliotibial tract
15) posterior superior iliac spine (PSIS)
16) sacrum
17) coccyx
18) gluteus maximus
19) gluteal cleft
20) gluteal fold
21) hamstrings
22) hamstring tendons
23) popliteal fossa

Bones & Bony Landmarks #1, p. 138

1) ilium, ischium, pubis - *p. 276*
2) sacrum, coccyx - *p. 276*
3) • female pelvis is broader for childbearing
    • wider iliac crest
    • larger pelvic "bowl"
    • greater distance between ischial tuberosities - *p. 276*
4) iliac crest - *p. 283*
5) posterior superior iliac spine (PSIS) - *p. 284*

6) ischial tuberosities - *p. 285*
7) greater trochanter - *p. 285*
8) iliac fossa - *p. 287*

Bones & Bony Landmarks #2, p. 139

1) hip
2) ilium
3) pubis
4) ischium
5) lumbar vertebra
6) sacroiliac joint
7) sacrum
8) sacrococcygeal joint
9) coccyx
10) coxal (hip) joint
11) femur
12) fifth lumbar vertebra
13) posterior superior iliac spine (PSIS)
14) medial sacral crest
15) greater trochanter
16) lesser trochanter
17) gluteal tuberosity
18) ischial tuberosity
19) obturator foramen

Hip, p. 140

1) iliac crest
2) iliac fossa
3) anterior superior iliac spine (ASIS)
4) anterior inferior iliac spine (AIIS)
5) pectineal line
6) superior ramus of the pubis
7) pubic tubercle
8) symphyseal surface
9) inferior ramus of pubis
10) posterior superior iliac spine (PSIS)
11) posterior inferior iliac spine (PIIS)
12) greater sciatic notch
13) ischial spine
14) lesser sciatic notch
15) obturator foramen
16) ischial tuberosity
17) ramus of the ischium
18) anterior gluteal line
19) posterior gluteal line
20) posterior superior iliac spine (PSIS)
21) inferior gluteal line
22) posterior inferior iliac spine (PIIS)
23) greater sciatic notch
24) ischial spine
25) lesser sciatic notch
26) obturator foramen
27) ischial tuberosity

28) iliac crest
29) iliac tubercle
30) anterior superior iliac spine (ASIS)
31) anterior inferior iliac spine (AIIS)
32) acetabulum
33) superior ramus of the pubis
34) pubic tubercle
35) inferior ramus of the pubis

Pelvis & Sacrum, p. 141

1) posterior superior iliac spine (PSIS)
2) posterior inferior iliac spine (PIIS)
3) ischial spine
4) ischial tuberosity
5) obturator foramen
6) ramus of ischium
7) inferior ramus of pubis
8) pubic symphysis
9) sacrum
10) gluteal surface of ilium
11) coccyx
12) acetabulum

Femur, p. 142

1) greater trochanter
2) patellar surface
3) lateral epicondyle
4) lateral condyle
5) head
6) fovea of head
7) neck
8) lesser trochanter
9) intertrochanteric line
10) shaft
11) adductor tubercle
12) medial epicondyle
13) medial condyle
14) head
15) neck
16) intertrochanteric crest
17) lesser trochanter
18) pectineal line
19) medial lip of linea aspera
20) lateral lip of linea aspera
21) adductor tubercle
22) medial epicondyle
23) medial condyle
24) greater trochanter
25) trochanteric fossa
26) gluteal tuberosity
27) intercondylar fossa
28) lateral epicondyle
29) lateral condyle

Bones & Bony Landmarks #3, p. 143
1) sacrum, coccyx - *p. 288, 289*
2) medial sacral crest - *p. 288*
3) gluteal cleft - *p. 289*
4) sacroiliac - *p. 289*
5) flex partner's knee to 90 degrees and rotate the hip laterally and medially - *p. 289*
6) gluteal tuberosity - *p. 290*
7) • explain what you are doing
   • ask permission
   • use partner's hand to palpate with your hand guiding on top - *p. 291*
8) pubic tubercles - *p. 291*
9) pectineus - *p. 292*
10) pubic crest, ischial tuberosity - *p. 292*
11) supine, with your flexed knee under your partner's knee - *p. 292*
12) gluteal fold - *p. 293*

Muscles of Pelvis & Thigh #1, p. 144
1) psoas major
2) psoas minor
3) iliacus
4) inguinal ligament
5) tensor fasciae latae
6) sartorius
7) iliotibial tract
8) rectus femoris
9) vastus lateralis
10) vastus medialis
11) pectineus
12) adductor longus
13) gracilis

Muscles of Pelvis & Thigh #2, p. 145
1) gracilis
2) adductor magnus
3) semitendinosus
4) semimembranosus
5) gluteus medius
6) tensor fasciae latae
7) gluteus maximus
8) iliotibial tract
9) biceps femoris (long head)
10) biceps femoris (short head)

Muscles of Pelvis & Thigh #3, p. 146
1) adductor longus
2) gracilis
3) adductor magnus
4) semimembranosus
5) semitendinosus
6) sartorius

7) vastus medialis
8) tendon of semitendinosus
9) pes anserinus tendon

Muscles of Pelvis & Thigh #4, p. 147
1) gluteus maximus
2) gluteus medius
3) gluteal fascia
4) tensor fasciae latae
5) sartorius
6) rectus femoris
7) iliotibial tract
8) vastus lateralis
9) biceps femoris (long head)
10) biceps femoris (short head)

Color the Muscles #1-4, p. 148-151

Muscles and Movements #1, p. 152
1) coxal
2) extension of hip
3) biceps femoris
   adductor magnus (posterior fibers)
4) rectus femoris
5) adduction of hip
6) gracilis
   gluteus maximus (lower fibers)
   iliacus
7) tensor fasciae latae
8) medial rotation of flexed knee
9) semitendinosus
   semimembranosus
   sartorius
   popliteus
10) biceps femoris

Muscles and Movements #2, p. 153
1) tibiofemoral
2) extension of knee
3) vastus lateralis
   vastus medialis
   vastus intermedius
4) gracilis
   gastrocnemius
5) abduction of hip
6) gluteus maximus (all fibers)
   gluteus medius (all fibers)
   gluteus minimus
7) pectineus
   psoas major
8) medial rotation of hip
9) gluteus medius (anterior fibers)
   gluteus minimus
   gracilis
   pectineus
10) biceps femoris

Muscles and Movements #3, p. 154
1) tibiofemoral
2) flexion of knee
3) biceps femoris
   gracilis
   gastrocnemius
4) rectus femoris
5) lateral (external) rotation of hip
6) piriformis
   psoas major
   iliacus
7) adductor magnus
   adductor longus
   adductor brevis
8) lateral rotation of flexed knee
9) biceps femoris
10) semitendinosus
   semimembranosus
   sartorius
11) flexion of hip
12) tensor fasciae latae
   sartorius
13) gluteus maximus (all fibers)
   gluteus medius (posterior fibers)

What's the Muscle? #1, p. 155
1) gluteus maximus
2) adductor brevis
3) vastus intermedius
4) obturator externus
5) semitendinosus
6) iliacus
7) sartorius
8) gemellus superior
9) pectineus

What's the Muscle? #2, p. 156
1) piriformis
2) vastus intermedius
3) adductor magnus
4) adductor longus
5) psoas minor
6) tensor fasciae latae
7) quadratus femoris
8) gluteus medius
9) semimembranosus

What's the Muscle? #3, p. 157
1) obturator internus
2) vastus medialis
3) gracilis
4) biceps femoris (long head)
5) gluteus minimus

Answer Pages

6) rectus femoris
7) psoas major
8) gemellus inferior

Muscle Group #1, p. 158
1) coxal (hip), tibiofemoral (knee)
   - *p. 294*
2) rectus femoris - *p. 300*
3) vastus lateralis - *p. 300*
4) AIIS, patella - *p. 303*
5) vastus medialis - *p. 304*
6) ischial tuberosity - *p. 305*
7) vastus lateralis, adductor magnus
   - *p. 305*
8) laterally - *p. 306*
9) semitendinosus
   - *p. 305, diagram 6.61*

Muscle Group #1, p. 159

Muscle	O	I
biceps femoris	4	7
rectus femoris	2	10
semimembranosus	3	8
semitendinosus	3	9
vastus intermedius	1	10
vastus lateralis	5	10
vastus medialis	6	10

11) lengthen
12) lengthen
13) shorten
14) shorten
15) shorten
16) lengthen, shorten

Muscle Group #2, p. 160
1) gluteus maximus - *p. 309*
2) gluteus medius - *p. 309*
3) gluteus maximus - *p. 311*
4) gluteus medius - *p. 312*
5) "abduct your hip" - *p. 312*
6) superior ramus of the pubis, ischial tuberosity - *p. 313*
7) adductor magnus - *p. 313*
8) knee - *p. 313*
9) adduct and medially rotate the hip
   - *p. 314*
10) pubic tubercle - *p. 316*
11) pectineus - *p. 317*
12) adductor magnus - *p. 317*

Muscle Group #2, p. 161

Muscle	O	I
adductor brevis	4	14
adductor longus	7	12
adductor magnus	6	13
gluteus maximus	1	10
gluteus medius	3	11
gluteus minimus	2	9
gracilis	5	16
pectineus	8	15

17) lengthen
18) shorten
19) shorten
20) lengthen
21) lengthen
22) lengthen
23) shorten
24) lengthen

Muscle Group #3, p. 162
1) tensor fasciae latae - *p. 318*
2) iliotibial tract - *p. 318*
3) "medially rotate your hip" - *p. 319*
4) sartorius - *p. 320*
5) femoral - *p. 320*
6) semitendinosus, gracilis, sartorius
   - *p. 321*
7) piriformis - *p. 322*
8) coccyx, PSIS, greater trochanter
   - *p. 324*
9) quadratus femoris - *p. 325*
10) psoas major - *p. 326*
11) ASIS, navel - *p. 328*
12) • explain what you are doing
    • communicate with your partner
    • slowly remove your hands if your partner feels unsafe or uncomfortable
    • have client take a deep breath and compress on their exhale
    • use small circles as you compress
    • be mindful of the pulse of the abdominal aorta and reposition laterally if you feel it - *p. 328*
13) "flex your hip ever so slightly"
    - *p. 328*

Muscle Group #3, p. 163

Muscle	O	I
gemellus inferior	8	20
gemellus superior	7	20
iliacus	6	14
obturator externus	11	19
obturator internus	10	15
piriformis	2	12
psoas major	4	14
psoas minor	3	18
quadratus femoris	9	16
sartorius	1	17
tensor fasciae latae	5	13

Muscle Group #3, p. 164
1) shorten
2) lengthen
3) lengthen
4) shorten
5) lengthen
6) shorten
7) shorten
8) shorten
9) lengthen
10) shorten

Other Structures #1, p. 165
1) inguinal ligament
2) sartorius
3) adductor longus
4) femoral nerve
5) femoral artery
6) femoral vein
7) inguinal ligament
8) adductor longus
9) inguinal lymph nodes
10) great saphenous vein
11) sartorius

Joints & Ligaments #1, p. 166
1) anterior longitudinal ligament
2) iliolumbar ligament
3) anterior sacroiliac ligament
4) sacrotuberous ligament
5) inguinal ligament
6) sacrospinous ligament
7) pubic symphysis
8) supraspinous ligament
9) iliolumbar ligament
10) posterior sacroiliac ligaments
11) sacrotuberous ligament
12) hamstrings tendon
13) posterior sacrococcygeal ligaments
14) sacrospinous ligament

Joints & Ligaments #2, p. 167
1) posterior sacroiliac ligaments
2) sacrotuberous ligament
3) sacrospinous ligament
4) articular capsule of coxal joint

5) tendon of rectus femoris (cut)
6) acetabulum
7) lunate surface of acetabulum
8) round ligament (ligamentum capitis femoris - cut)
9) obturator membrane
10) anterior sacroiliac ligament
11) sacrospinous ligament
12) sacrotuberous ligament
13) obturator membrane
14) pubic symphysis

Coxal Joint, p. 168
1) iliofemoral ligament
2) pubofemoral ligament
3) femur
4) iliofemoral ligament
5) ischiofemoral ligament
6) zona orbicularis
7) articular cartilage
8) lunate surface of acetabulum
9) acetabular labrum
10) transverse acetabular ligament
11) round ligament (ligamentum capitis femoris - cut)

Other Structures #2, p. 169
1) ASIS, pubic tubercle - *p. 333*
2) femoral artery, femoral nerve, femoral vein - *p. 333*
3) between ASIS and pubic tubercle, just distal to the inguinal ligament - *p. 333*
4) sacrotuberous ligament - *p. 334*
5) sacroiliac - *p. 334*
6) iliolumbar - *p. 335*
7) sciatic nerve - *p. 335*
8) trochanteric bursa - *p. 336*

✦ Leg & Foot

Topographical Views, p. 171
1) popliteal fossa
2) patella
3) tibial tuberosity
4) pes anserinus attachment site
5) gastrocnemius
6) tibialis anterior
7) shaft of the tibia
8) calcaneal tendon
9) lateral malleolus
10) medial malleolus
11) tibialis anterior tendon

12) tibialis anterior tendon
13) extensor hallucis longus tendon
14) extensor digitorum longus tendons

Bones & Bony Landmarks of Knee & Leg, p. 172
1) tibiofemoral - *p. 340*
2) flexed - *p. 340*
3) tibia, fibula - *p. 340*
4) proximal tibia, femoral condyles - *p. 344*
5) tibial tuberosity - *p. 344*
6) patellar ligament - *p. 301, 344*
7) biceps femoris, soleus, fibular collateral ligament - *p. 345*
8) the edges - *p. 345*
9) sartorius, gracilis, semitendinosus - *p. 346*
10) edges of femoral condyles - *p. 346*
11) iliotibial tract - *p. 347*
12) adductor tubercle, adductor magnus - *p. 347*

Bones of Knee, Leg & Foot, p. 173
1) femur
2) patella
3) tibia
4) fibula
5) talus
6) tarsals
7) metatarsals
8) phalanges
9) medial and lateral intercondylar tubercles
10) lateral condyle
11) head of the fibula
12) lateral malleolus
13) medial condyle
14) tibial tuberosity
15) soleal line
16) medial malleolus
17) medial malleolus
18) fossa of lateral malleolus
19) lateral condyle
20) lateral malleolus

Bony Landmarks of Knee and Leg, p. 174
1) tibial tuberosity
2) adductor tubercle
3) medial epicondyle
4) medial condyle
5) tibial plateau
6) pes anserinus attachment site

7) lateral epicondyle
8) lateral condyle
9) tibial plateau
10) tibial tubercle
11) head of the fibula
12) tibial tuberosity
13) shaft of the tibia

Bones of Foot, p. 175
1) calcaneus
2) talus
3) cuboid
4) navicular
5) lateral, middle and medial cuneiforms
6) metatarsals
7) phalanges
8) phalanges
9) sesamoid bones
10) metatarsals
11) lateral, middle and medial cuneiforms
12) navicular
13) cuboid
14) talus
15) calcaneus

Bones & Bony Landmarks of Foot #1, p. 176
1) lateral and middle cuneiforms
2) metatarsals
3) base
4) shaft
5) head
6) tuberosity of fifth metatarsal
7) cuboid
8) peroneal trochlea
9) calcaneus
10) talus
11) navicular
12) base of first metatarsal
13) trochlea of the talus
14) talus
15) medial tubercle of talus
16) sustentaculum tali
17) calcaneus
18) tuberosity of calcaneus
19) head of the talus
20) navicular tubercle
21) medial cuneiform
22) head
23) shaft
24) base
25) phalanges

Calcaneus & Talus, p. 177
1) body
2) peroneal trochlea
3) groove for peroneus longus tendon
4) articular surfaces for talus
5) tuberosity
6) sustentaculum tali
7) groove for flexor hallucis longus tendon
8) trochlea
9) neck
10) head
11) lateral tubercle
12) lateral process
13) tarsal sinus
14) trochlea
15) neck
16) head
17) medial tubercle

Bones & Bony Landmarks of Foot #2, p. 178
1) calcaneus, talus - *p. 348*
2) dorsal - *p. 348*
3) lateral malleolus - *p. 351*
4) invert the foot - *p. 351*
5) distal, one inch - *p. 353*
6) medial malleolus, navicular tubercle - *p. 354*
7) invert and plantar flex - *p. 355*
8) medial cuneiform - *p. 356*
9) dorsal and medial surfaces - *p. 356*
10) proximal interphalangeal, distal interphalangeal - *p. 356*
11) peroneus brevis - *p. 357*
12) tibialis anterior - *p. 358*
13) tuberosity of fifth metatarsal - *p. 359*
14) tuberosity of fifth metatarsal, lateral malleolus - *p. 359*

Muscles of Leg & Foot #1, p. 179
1) plantaris
2) gastrocnemius
3) soleus
4) calcaneal tendon
5) flexor tendons
6) peroneal tendons
7) superior peroneal retinaculum
8) flexor retinaculum
9) gastrocnemius (cut)
10) plantaris

11) popliteus
12) soleus
13) gastrocnemius (cut)
14) calcaneal tendon

Muscles of Leg & Foot #2, p. 180
1) peroneus longus
2) tibialis anterior
3) gastrocnemius
4) soleus
5) extensor digitorum longus
6) peroneus brevis
7) peroneus longus
8) tibialis anterior
9) gastrocnemius
10) soleus
11) peroneus brevis
12) extensor digitorum longus
13) extensor hallucis longus

Muscles of Leg & Foot #3, p. 181
1) tibialis anterior
2) extensor hallucis longus
3) extensor digitorum longus
4) peroneus longus
5) peroneus brevis
6) flexor hallucis longus
7) tibialis posterior
8) flexor digitorum longus
9) soleus
10) calcaneal tendon

Color the Muscles #1-2, p. 182-183

Muscles and Movements #1, p. 184
1) talocrural
2) dorsiflexion of ankle
3) tibialis anterior
   extensor digitorum longus
   extensor hallucis longus
4) flexor digitorum longus (weak)
   flexor hallucis longus (weak)
5) eversion of foot
6) peroneus longus
   peroneus brevis
7) tibialis anterior
   tibialis posterior
8) flexion of toes
9) flexor digitorum longus
   flexor digitorum brevis
   flexor digiti minimi (5th)
10) lumbricals

Muscles and Movements #2, p. 185
1) metacarpophalangeal, proximal interphalangeal, distal interphalangeal
2) extension of toes
3) extensor digitorum longus
   extensor digitorum brevis (2nd - 4th)
   lumbricals
4) flexor digitorum longus
   flexor digitorum brevis
   flexor digiti minimi (5th)
5) inversion of foot
6) tibialis anterior
   tibialis posterior
   flexor digitorum longus
   flexor hallucis longus
7) extensor digitorum longus
8) plantar flexion of ankle
9) soleus
   tibialis posterior
10) extensor digitorum longus
   extensor hallucis longus

What's the Muscle? #1, p. 186
1) popliteus
2) extensor hallucis longus
3) flexor digitorum brevis
4) extensor digitorum longus
5) soleus
6) gastrocnemius
7) tibialis posterior
8) abductor digiti minimi

What's the Muscle? #2, p. 187
1) extensor digitorum brevis
2) plantaris
3) peroneus longus
4) abductor hallucis
5) flexor hallucis longus
6) tibialis anterior
7) flexor digitorum longus
8) peroneus brevis

Muscle Group #1, p. 188
1) gastrocnemius, soleus - *p. 364*
2) calcaneal tendon - *p. 364*
3) stand on his toes - *p. 365*
4) medial - *p. 365*
5) medially, shaft of the tibia - *p. 366*
6) plantaris - *p. 367*
7) inch, oblique - *p. 367*
8) popliteus - *p. 368*

9) unlocking the joint - "the key which unlocks the knee" - *p. 368*
10) soleus, gastrocnemius - *p. 368*
11) lateral, extensor digitorum longus, soleus - *p. 369*
12) head of the fibula, lateral malleolus - *p. 370*
13) evert the foot - *p. 370*

Muscle Group #1, p. 189

Muscle	O	I
gastrocnemius	4	8
peroneus brevis	1	10
peroneus longus	5	7
plantaris	3	8
popliteus	2	9
soleus	6	8

11) lengthen
12) lengthen
13) lengthen
14) shorten

Muscle Group #2, p. 190
1) tibial shaft - *p. 371*
2) dorsiflex or invert the foot - *p. 372*
3) extensor retinaculum - *p. 371, 373*
4) tibial shaft, edge of the soleus/calcaneal tendon - *p. 374*
5) tibialis posterior
   flexor digitorum longus
   tibial artery
   tibial nerve
   flexor hallucis longus - *p. 376*
6) wiggle all his toes - *p. 376*
7) extensor digitorum brevis - *p. 377*
8) plantar aponeurosis - *p. 377*
9) extensor digitorum longus - *p. 378*
10) plantar surface of the heel, second through fifth toes - *p. 378*
11) flex the first toe - *p. 379*
12) calcaneus, head of the first metatarsal, head of the fifth metatarsal - *p. 379*

Muscle Group #2, p. 191

Muscle	O	I
extensor digitorum longus	1	10
extensor hallucis longus	3	7
flexor digitorum longus	5	8
flexor hallucis longus	4	7
tibialis anterior	2	9
tibialis posterior	6	11

12) shorten
13) lengthen
14) shorten
15) lengthen

Tibiofemoral Joint, p. 192
1) femur
2) anterior cruciate ligament
3) lateral meniscus
4) fibular collateral ligament
5) anterior ligament of head of the fibula
6) fibula
7) posterior cruciate ligament
8) tibial collateral ligament
9) medial meniscus
10) transverse ligament of knee
11) tibia
12) patellar ligament (cut)
13) posterior meniscofemoral ligament
14) posterior cruciate ligament
15) anterior cruciate ligament
16) fibular collateral ligament
17) popliteus tendon (cut)
18) lateral meniscus
19) posterior ligament of head of the fibula
20) medial meniscus
21) tibial collateral ligament

Tibiofemoral & Tibiofibular Joints, p. 193
1) anterior cruciate ligament (cut)
2) lateral meniscus
3) posterior meniscofemoral ligament (cut)
4) posterior cruciate ligament (cut)
5) medial meniscus
6) iliotibial tract (cut)
7) fibular collateral ligament (cut)
8) biceps femoris tendon (cut)
9) anterior ligament of head of fibula
10) interosseous membrane
11) fibula
12) anterior tibiofibular ligament
13) anterior talofibular ligament (cut)
14) cruciate ligaments (cut)
15) tibial collateral ligament (cut)
16) patellar ligament (cut)
17) tibia

Other Structures of Knee, p. 194
1) quadriceps femoris tendon
2) femur
3) patella
4) prepatellar bursa
5) patellar ligament
6) subcutaneous infrapatellar bursa
7) deep infrapatellar bursa
8) tibia
9) hamstrings
10) popliteal artery and vein
11) tibial nerve
12) common peroneal nerve
13) gastrocnemius
14) lesser saphenous vein

Talocrural Joint, p. 195
1) posterior tibiofibular ligament
2) lateral malleolus
3) anterior tibiofibular ligament
4) anterior talofibular ligament
5) posterior talofibular ligament
6) calcaneofibular ligament
7) deltoid ligament
8) posterior tibiotalar ligament
9) tibiocalcaneal ligament
10) anterior tibiotalar ligament
11) tibionavicular ligament
12) navicular
13) sustentaculum tali
14) medial malleolus

Talocrural & Talotarsal Joints, p. 196
1) tibia
2) talus
3) deltoid ligament
4) fibula
5) posterior tibiofibular ligament
6) posterior talofibular ligament
7) calcaneofibular ligament
8) posterior talocalcaneal ligament
9) calcaneus
10) posterior talocalcaneal ligament
11) talonavicular ligament
12) talus
13) navicular
14) lateral talocalcaneal ligament
15) interosseous talocalcaneal ligament

Ligaments of Foot, p. 197

1) plantar metatarsal ligaments
2) long plantar ligament
3) plantar calcaneocuboid (short plantar) ligament
4) plantar cuboideonavicular ligament
5) navicular
6) plantar calcaneonavicular (spring) ligament
7) plantar calcaneocuboid (short plantar) ligament
8) plantar calcaneonavicular (spring) ligament
9) long plantar ligament
10) dorsal cuneonavicular ligaments
11) dorsal intercuneiform ligaments
12) dorsal cuneocuboid ligament
13) dorsal cuboideonavicular ligament
14) bifurcate ligament
15) dorsal calcaneocuboid ligaments

Other Structures of Knee, Leg & Foot, p. 198

1) lateral epicondyle of femur, head of the fibula - *p. 384*
2) medial - *p. 384*
3) weight distribution, friction reduction - *p. 385*
4) medially - *p. 385*
5) prepatellar bursa - *p. 386*
6) medial, lateral, posterior - *p. 387*
7) flex and extend the toes - *p. 393*
8) talus, sustentaculum tali, navicular - *p. 391*
9) sustentaculum tali, navicular tubercle, tibialis posterior tendon - *p. 391*
10) fibers are superficial and perpendicular - *p. 392*
11) medial malleolus, medial calcaneus - *p. 393*
12) inferior, posterior - *p. 392, 393*
13) dorsalis pedis - *p. 394*
14) calcaneal tendon, overlying skin - *p. 394*